Powerwatch

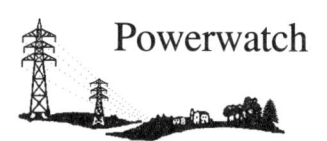

We find that this book answers most people's questions about the use of electrical appliances in their home & environment.

Call our premium rate* **helpline number 0897 100 800** for personal advice and further information about specific issue including surveys, reports, presentations and training.
(*Premium rate calls are charged at £1.50/minute)

We also offer a consultancy service.

We use electrical appliances a lot of the time in our own homes, often without considering the electromagnetic fields that are generated and that research is beginning to show may affect us adversely in subtle ways. This book has been written to help you find ways of living safely with the things you want to use, helping you to decide what you *need* and what you can begin to manage without.

We would like to thank Ruth and Graham for their patience in putting up with our preoccupations and time pressures.

The booklet has been written by Alasdair and Jean Philips.

This booklet is dedicated to all people who are choosing to become responsible for their own health and well-being. May the Force be with you!

ISBN 1-897-761-198

**Published by Green Audit Books,
Green Audit (Wales) Ltd
Aberystwyth**

This Book © 1999 by Alasdair & Jean Philips

Extra copies may be obtained, by post only, from
A & J Philips at
2 Tower Road, Sutton, Ely, Cambs., CB6 2QA
at a cost of £8.50 including p&p (U.K. only)
(Cheques payable to A & J Philips, please)

CONTENTS

Chapter 1. General Introduction — 1
Electric and Magnetic fields
A general overview of EMFs
Possible health effects
The biology, including Melatonin

Chapter 2. Your Home — 12
A tour around your home
EMF exposure in different rooms
Precautions you can take

Chapter 3. Around and About — 41
Cars
Mobile Phones & masts
Substations, pylons & cables

Chapter 4. Special Needs — 52
Hearing aids, personal alarms
Lifts, stairlifts & wheelchairs

Chapter 5. Appliance List — 56
An alphabetical list of appliances - problems & precautions

Chapter 6. Wiring and Reducing Fields — 96
Where elevated fields come from within the house
Prevention and cure of common problems in layperson's terms

Chapter 7. Protection Devices — 107
Gizmos, some of which might actually work!

Chapter 8. Useful Information — 119
Names, addresses, websites, and further reading

Appendices — 123
One: *Unit conversion table*
Two: *Aluminium foil Screening diagram*

CHAPTER ONE
GENERAL INTRODUCTION

In the course of the twentieth century, we have been increasingly exposed to equipment that uses electricity. We are now surrounded by electric and magnetic fields (EMFs) from our mains electricity supply millions of times higher than those experienced by our ancestors 100 years ago.

Indeed it is quite surprising when we look back to see just how recently we started to surround ourselves with these unnatural vibrations. Although limited radio telegraphy had been around since the start of the century, it wasn't until 1920 that the Marconi Company began experimental speech transmission from their Chelmsford factory on a very long wavelength of 2,750 metres.

It was 14th November 1922 when the BBC started broadcasting in London with station "2LO", to be joined the next day by "2ZY" in Manchester and "5IT" in Birmingham. Less than 80 years ago we were surrounded by virtually no radio-frequency or microwave radiation. Much of the United Kingdom still did not have an electricity supply, and in those areas which did, some were 'direct current' and did not vibrate many times every second. The village in Cambridgeshire where we live did not receive an electricity supply until 1939.

The real growth of commercial radio broadcasting started in the early 1930s. In December 1932 the 'Wireless Constructor' was reporting: *"Every week one reads of some station planning to radiate enormous power, some fiddling little continental will suddenly develop into an overpowering giant"* and warns that unless people could screen out the unwanted signals **"you may find yourself in the position of a paralysed man watching the rising of a tide which will ultimately drown him."** Prophetic words?

When we are born, it is usually in a hospital, which is full of high-tech electrically operated machinery.

Very few homes are without labour-saving devices and machinery to entertain us and enliven our leisure time.

Outside, our gardens echo to the sounds of mowers, and the streets (not to mention buses and trains!) resound to the ring of mobile phones! Cars are the most used form of personal transport. Radio & TV and mobile phone masts, certainly the latter, are springing up like new age forests.

At school, children at increasingly young ages are learning to use computer technology; many youngsters being far more flexible and adept at picking up the new knowledge than their parents. Cases of childhood RSI have been reported.

At work photocopiers, faxes, printers, computers, etc. surround us.

Even during our leisure and holiday time we are exposed to electrical equipment in cars, buses, aeroplanes, and when we get to our destination, in concerts, theatres, raves, bowling alleys, etc. In many ways we do not know what effect this may be having on our health.

Human bodies have not been exposed to this level of ambient electrical energy before. It's almost impossible to find out whether long-term health effects are *caused* by *specific* environmental pollutants when most people are exposed most of the time.

Epidemiology (the study of illnesses in the general population) is good at identifying isolated and acute disease conditions. However, results are often misleading and inaccurate when applied to widespread, low-level chronic conditions. So it is possible that most societies have been suffering from the effects of rising long-term background electromagnetic exposure for the last few generations. No one has yet scientifically "proved" the link; although certain illnesses have been associated with exposure to electromagnetic radiation many times in different studies and different countries. This is particularly true of some cancers; especially childhood leukaemia and breast cancer, as well as Alzheimer's disease and depression.

It is difficult to separate out different pollutants where heavy-metals, arsenic, pesticides, etc. in the water supply have been lightly poisoning whole communities for generations. It often takes decades after the first suspicion of a problem for the authorities to accept that there is something to investigate. We might remember the examples of smoking, asbestos, CJD etc. We are all guineapigs in the grand experiment. It is interesting to note that we are also experiencing many new health problems (ME & HIV, to name but two); viruses are known to be mutating, and bacteria are becoming resistant to antibiotics.

The diagnosis of acute lymphoblastic leukaemia (ALL), the commonest form of childhood leukaemia, now peaks between the ages of one and six years. The peak first appeared in the 1930's and the number of children developing this illness is continuing to rise. The rise may be partly due to the fact that children with immune systems that weren't working properly, began to live long enough to develop the disease. The 1930's was also when many houses were first linked to the network of electricity distribution. Even if there is a connection between these two events, it is unlikely to be a straightforward cause-effect relationship. However some research by Lai & Singh in 1996 shows the ability of electromagnetic radiation to affect the actual structure of DNA, the building blocks of life.

At a biological level, our bodies communicate chemically and electrically at intercellular (between different cells) and intracellular (within the same cell) levels. It is possible that our exposure to electric and magnetic fields during our daily activities may be preventing our bodies from being in the best state of health. Many recent laboratory studies have shown that exposure to electromagnetic fields negatively affect cellular processes. Professor Russel Reiter states that "reduction of melatonin at night increases a cell's vulnerability to alteration by carcinogenic agents".

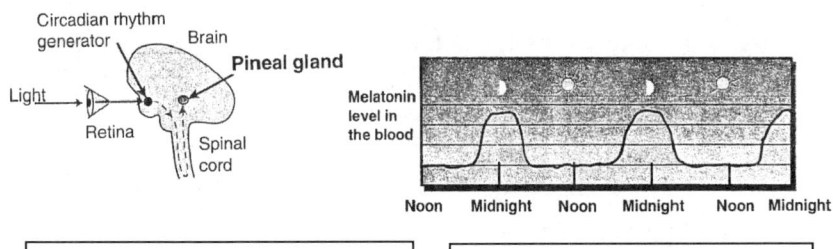

Light regulates melatonin secretion by the pineal gland. It is also affected by EMFs.	Melatonin levels are low during the day and should rise at night when it is dark.

Melatonin plays a key part in helping the body repair itself, and thus reject pre-cancerous cells. It is produced by the pineal gland as it synthesises the chemical serotonin. This mainly happens at night, the pineal gland being "switched on" by dark conditions. <u>Melatonin is also less effective in its action when exposed to EMFs.</u> This is one of the reasons that it is important to have lower electromagnetic field levels in bedrooms.

Constant EMF exposure may actually promote illnesses that otherwise a healthy body would have easily resisted. Melatonin is found to be low in people suffering from clinical depression. We don't know for certain why this is. One GP in the West Midlands found a connection that was statistically significant between people suffering from depression and those attempting suicide and how near they lived to high voltage pylons and cables giving off high EMFs for 24 hours a day.

Important cellular processes that play a central role in the development of the immune system, are adversely affected by EMFs. Experiments have shown links between EMFs and fatigue, headaches, slower reaction times, irregular heartbeat and altered brain waves.

However, it is very difficult these days to imagine living in a house without electricity. Some years ago, we visited friends who were not connected to the mains electricity, but relied on a generator for their power. It had taken some time for them to get used to only using the things which needed electricity at times when the generator made it available to them. Hot water (except what was boiled on the solid-fuel Aga), washing, ironing, watching television, listening to music, all had to be carefully planned for. Oil lamps produced a beautiful soft light, but detailed work like reading, writing, or sewing was more difficult, especially in winter when natural light is limited. The Centre for Alternative Technology in Machynlleth, Wales, uses alternative sources of energy, (solar and wind mainly), and the people living there use electricity on a rota basis. Most of us feel that we do not want to choose this self-limiting path. Some of us will remember the frustrations and dangers of electricity rationing during the weeks of the miners' strike in the 1970's. Until and unless the price of electricity causes us to change our consumption because of cost implications, we wish to have constant access to electricity for our everyday use.

This book has been written to help you to become more aware of the sea of electric and magnetic radiation you are bathed in, and how to minimise your exposure whilst still using the equipment you want to use. With this information you can reduce the possibilities of adverse health risks associated with the use of electricity. Professor Morgan, of Carnegie Mellon University, says that although EMFs *may* pose no risk, most experts he has talked to give him odds somewhere between 10% and 60% that within the next decade it will become clear that they *do*. Meanwhile, he suggests, taking "prudent avoidance" sounds like a sensible precaution.

In 1998 a scientific committee of the U.S. National Institute of Environmental Health Services concluded that power frequency EMFs were 'possible human carcinogens'. In 1999 in the final report to Congress, the NIEHS Director endorsed a policy of *"prudent avoidance"*, or taking simple and inexpensive steps to limit exposures. The Government of Sweden backed prudent avoidance of power frequency health risks in 1995. The idea was first put forward by the Congressional Office of Technology Assessment in 1989.

Children are more susceptible to influences from EMFs because their cells are multiplying much more rapidly as they grow and are therefore more prone to damage from external, or internal sources.

More and more people are developing a syndrome called Electrical Sensitivity. They become so sensitive to electrical stimulation that their lives can, in extreme cases, become restricted to a non-electrical environment. Obviously, this has implications for home life, working ability, and overall well-being. Some Swedish companies have produced 'low EMF rooms' so that their ES people can continue to work. Once sensitised, there is very little that can be done to "cure" the condition. Changes can be made that make it liveable with, and more bearable, but the important thing is to try and avoid its developing in the first place. Sometimes electrical sensitivity develops after exposure to hazardous chemicals, and is further complicated by MCS (Multiple Chemical Sensitivity). The condition is often not recognised by the medical profession, and sufferers may be referred to the Psychiatric services for treatment.

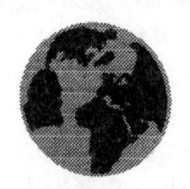

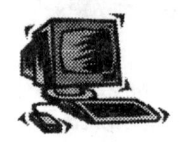

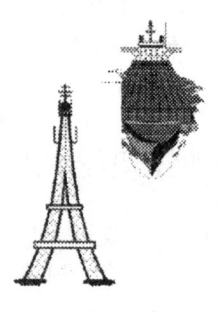

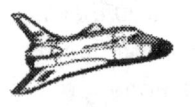

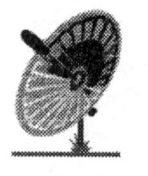

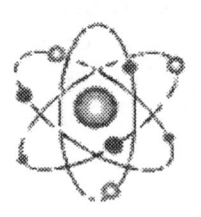

Frequency	Typical use	Wavelength
1 Hz	Earth and planetary signals	300,000 km
10 Hz	Brain waves	30,000 km
100 Hz	**50 Hz mains electricity**	3,000 km
1 kHz		300 km
10 kHz		30 km
100 kHz	Radio-navigation	3 km
1 MHz	Long Wave broadcasting
Medium Wave broadcasting	300 metres
10 MHz	Short Wave radio stations
CB radio	30 metres
100 MHz	**VHF FM** radio stations
Police and Aircraft radio
TV broadcasting	3 metres
1 GHz	**Mobile phones
Microwave ovens**
Radar, Satellite	30 cm
10 GHz	Fixed microwave links
experimental microwave	3 cm
100 GHz	work - radar
and imaging	3 mm
1 THz	Atomic resonances	0.3 mm
10 THz		30 µm
100 THz	Infra Red
Visible Light
Ultra Violet	3 µm
1000 THz	**X**-rays
Gamma rays	300 nm
300 pm
300 fm

The continuous electromagnetic spectrum

Most of the regulations concerning exposure to electromagnetic radiation refer to high level, short-term exposure. These regulations are imposed by the government, which in turn, is advised by the National Radiological Protection Board (NRPB). The guidelines were laid down primarily because of concerns to do with ionising radiation (e.g. ultra violet light and nuclear radiation). Acute effects from 'non-ionising' EMFs include interference with our central nervous system at low frequencies and heating of body tissue at radiofrequencies. The regulations also protect against direct electric shock and spark discharges.

It must be remembered that ALL items connected to the mains electricity supply will give off both electric and magnetic fields when working. At low frequencies (usually the frequency of our mains electricity supply which vibrates 50 times every second), the electric and magnetic components of the fields are not related mathematically to each other, and so it is necessary to think about them separately.

Electrical appliances may also give off radio-frequency and microwave radiation. At these high frequencies they 'radiate' around the world as radiowaves and can travel long distances.

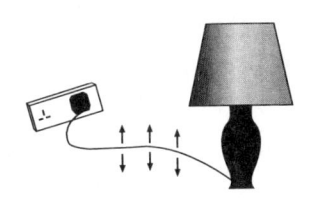

When an electrical appliance is plugged in at a wall socket, it will give off an electric field, even when it is switched off at the appliance. The further you are away from an appliance, the weaker the field will be, as electric fields decrease with distance. The field is produced by the voltage fed to the appliance from the mains. It is measured in volts per metre (V/m) or in kilovolts per metre (kV/m). The NRPB (the Government advisory body) suggests that the average field level in the centre of a room is typically about 10 V/m. In practice, we would say that 20 V/m is more realistic in modern housing. In bedrooms, it should be no higher than 10 V/m, and ideally be zero. Electric fields rise rapidly towards most ceilings and light switches. Sockets give off electric fields unless they are metal-clad and the wires are in metal conduit. Electric fields may be shielded or weakened by walls, fences, growing plants etc. The electric field produced by an appliance in one room is unlikely to extend into a room the other side of the wall, although walls which may be slightly, almost undetectably, damp can become conductive. They can then pick up an electric field and re-radiate it over a large area. Commonly the field is picked up from an electric socket or light switch.

With careful design, it is possible to minimise EMFs from house wiring. This is dealt with in chapter 6.

A magnetic field is produced when a current flows along the wire to the appliance. Magnetic fields are measured in units of magnetic flux, nanotesla (nT) and microtesla (µT; 1000 nT = 1µT). In America it is measured in milliGauss (see Appendix 1). We will use nanotesla throughout, as we believe that changing scales can add confusion to this already complex subject. In living areas and especially sleeping areas, magnetic fields should be less than 200 nT, ideally less than 50 nT. The 'average' UK ambient power-frequency magnetic field in homes is around 40 nT. Average field levels tend to be higher in flats (50 - 80 nT). The magnetic field levels that research has shown are associated with adverse health problems are those higher than 200 nT. In bedrooms where people spend a long time without moving, their bodies repairing the damages of the day, we recommend that the fields should be no higher than 50 nT.

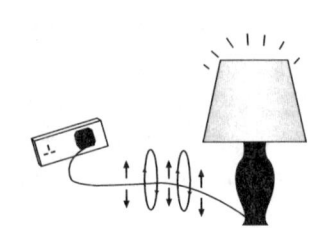

Field levels can vary considerably during a 24-hour period. To get an idea of the *maximum* normal level, it is necessary to measure them at a peak load time. The best time for this is 5.00 to 6.30 p.m. during the week. In cold winter weather, field levels can be up to three times higher than in hot weather, because of the extra demand for heating. Night-time field levels can be high if your house or surrounding houses use electric off-peak heating. This can happen in more rural areas, where there is no gas supply to provide one of the alternative forms of heating. This clearly will make a difference to the field levels in bedrooms.

Magnetic fields can *not* be easily shielded or weakened by most materials. Sometimes thick sheet steel can be used or a special metal called Mumetal. Both of these are very expensive to use. Practically, it is much better not to *create* high magnetic fields in the first place. In the home, this should be possible.

There are a significant number of houses where large magnetic fields are produced by unseen and un-noticed wiring faults. These are usually in the circuits that feed power around the 13A mains wall sockets (see Chapter 6). They can also exist in lighting circuits - especially where there are two switches which control the same light. All wiring is required by law to comply with the current IEE wiring regulations.

The only way to find out if your wiring is causing high magnetic fields is to carry out some loading tests when measuring the magnetic fields with a meter. Suitable meters, with full instructions as to how to use them, and how to make the loading tests referred to, can be hired from Powerwatch (See Chapter 8).

Houses can be wired to produce virtually no electric and magnetic fields in most areas of the living space. However, modern domestic wiring techniques tend to cause high electric fields and can also lead to unnecessarily high magnetic fields. It is most important to reduce the level of fields in bedrooms and in those rooms where children and people who are unwell for any reason, spend most time. These are the people at most risk of being affected by higher than normal fields.

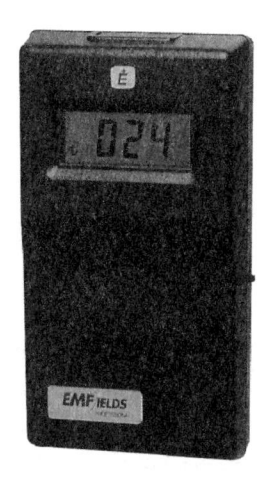

Some research done at Bristol University showed that the average number of hours spent in different rooms in the house was as follows:-

Room	Hours
Living room	5.2
Dining room	1.2
Kitchen	3.2
Bedroom	8.4
Bathroom	1.2
Study	0.6
Utility room	1.6

The times people spend in the rooms in *your* house may be quite different to the times shown above. The important thing is to minimise the fields in the rooms you and your family use most. This is especially true where you sit down, or lie down for long periods of time. This is usually in bedrooms and on specific chairs or settees in sitting rooms. Individuals may spend considerable time in front of TVs or computers.

Sources of high magnetic fields from outside, (e.g. high voltage powerlines or substations and their associated cabling,) are problems which you can do very little about. These are discussed in chapter 3.

Research into health effects has focused mainly on magnetic fields, since the initial work done by Wertheimer and Leeper in America in 1979. They began looking at our exposure to magnetic fields to see whether they were responsible for ill-health. It is only in the last few years that the importance of the electric field has also begun to be recognised. When high magnetic fields and high electric fields are found together, the incidence of health problems has been seen to go up from a factor of 2 or 3 to over 10 fold. It is not simply a matter of adding the two risks together.

It seems that damage from electromagnetic fields is both instantaneous and cumulative. A relatively small percentage of people seem to be far more sensitive to being affected by electromagnetic fields than others, probably for similar reasons that some people can smoke for years and not get lung cancer. This is probably due to a combination of genetic factors and exposure to chemicals and other environmental agents.

There are several reasons why you may fail to realise that EMFs are making you ill:
- If you move away from the EMF source there may be no obvious change for some considerable time.
- There can be a long latent period (5 to 15 years) before a well defined disease shows itself. Until that time the problem tends to produce many poorly defined symptoms.
- In general the medical profession does not recognise that any chronic adverse health effects can be caused by our use of electricity.

Although we recommend that it is always wise to minimise exposure to power frequency EMFs, we believe that high intensity short-term exposure is less likely to create health problems than long term lower level background exposure, especially in places where we sleep or sit for long periods of time. The published epidemiological evidence from most occupational studies show less health problems than from residential studies. One clear exception to this is industrial sewing machinists who sit for long periods in high fields from their machine motors - they have a statistically strong raised chance of developing Alzheimer's Disease or Amytropic Lateral Sclerosis.

At radio and microwave frequencies the evidence is accumulating that we also should try to minimise our exposure, instead of the current trend to use more and more radio based devices - e.g. mobile and cordless phones which emit microwave radiation. Remote gas and water meter reading and inbuilt car anti-collision radars are planned for introduction in the next few years and the 'wireless office' is already being installed - again using microwaves instead of wires to connect computers and phones.

Stanislav Smigielski monitored the Polish military personnel for over 15 years and found that those occupationally exposed to RF and microwave radiation were 14 times more likely to develop chronic leukaemia in their old age, 9 times more likely to develop acute leukaemia and 6 times more likely to develop Non-Hodgkin's Lymphoma (NHL). NHL incidence is rising steadily in Western countries for no known reason. The estimated average exposure levels of the people in Smigielski's study were only about 5 microwatts per square centimetre, a level which can be found near cellular phone base-stations, TV and radio transmitter masts, and are greatly exceeded next to mobile and cordless phones!

From looking at the evidence over many years, we are convinced that EMFs adversely affect some people and that it is wise for all of us to adopt the principle of keeping our EMF exposure *"as low as reasonably achievable"*. A way to reduce your cumulative exposure to EMFs is by choosing carefully what electrical appliances to surround you and your family with, and following the guidelines in this book.

CHAPTER TWO
YOUR HOME

In this chapter, we will take a tour around your home. We will point out some of the things to look for, to be wary of, to allow for in the positioning of furniture, and the carrying out of activities. Your home may not have all of the rooms mentioned, and in some houses the rooms are bigger than in others, allowing for the possibility of moving things around more easily. It is important to remember that magnetic fields go through walls and ceilings. **Any appliance that gives off high magnetic fields should not be within one metre of a chair that is sat in for long periods of time; or within one metre of the head of a bed.**

This applies when a chair or bedhead is immediately the other side of the wall to the appliance and the one metre guideline should be remembered in connection with the comments in this Chapter. The magnetic fields from some appliances which are near the ceiling (e.g. burglar alarms, fluorescent lights, etc.) may go through the ceiling and form areas of high EMFs in the room above.

The items in **bold** characters, are listed individually in Chapter 5. Chapter 5 is intended for reference purposes and contains much of the information included in this chapter in an easy-reference form. It sometimes contains extra, more detailed or more technical information. Chapter 2 is intended as a general overview guide.

We have had questions from people who experience a build-up of **static electricity** leading to shocks. We do not believe that this is good for the biological systems within the body. If you are troubled by static build-up, ensure you always wear natural fibre clothing (wool, cotton, linen, silk, etc.) and do not have carpets in your home that contain nylon or predominantly any synthetic fibre. It may be that the air in your house is too dry. Plenty of green plants can help humidify the air. Otherwise damp cloths hung on radiators can help. Static build-up when getting out of a car is covered in Chapter 3.

As an alternative to mains-driven appliances, we have been asked about the effects from **battery operated equipment.** Batteries do not give off high EMFs. However, they are not energy-efficient: manufacturing them uses 50 times more energy than they will ever produce. They usually contain mercury, cadmium, lithium and other toxic, non-biodegradable metals that can affect water supplies from land-fill. Rechargeable batteries should be used and then recycled if possible. It is better to consider your overall use of power-driven appliances, than merely to replace mains operated equipment with battery ones.

At the end of this chapter, you will find answers to some of the more general questions we have been asked. For example:- "Why do light bulbs fail regularly?"

But for now, we will begin the guided tour.

Let us start at the front door....

There could be two pieces of electrical equipment at, or immediately inside, the front door.

You might have an electric **door bell.** If this is battery operated then there will be no real EMF problems, although it might interfere with AM radio when the bell is ringing. If run from mains electricity then watch the position of the transformer which will be giving off magnetic fields.

You might have to quickly de-activate your **burglar alarm system.** This will have one **main control unit** and a number of **sensors** in different places throughout the house. The control units can have cheap transformers giving off high magnetic fields, or be unearthed and so give off high electric fields. If this is the case then all the wiring to the sensors and alarms will also be giving off high electric fields. Be careful if your unit is close to the ceiling – what is above? Remember that the main units are often meant to be tamper-proof, so DIY can have interesting results!

The sensors themselves do not give off significant EMFs, unless they are active microwave ones. Active microwave sensors usually give out low level microwaves all the time. It is a good idea to contact the company that installed them and make sure that they can be switched off when you are at home. Surprisingly many can't be switched off without a modification to the system controller!

Now we are inside the house, your electrical equipment may be in different places from those suggested. The guidelines given below apply to the equipment wherever it may be in your house.

Fire Alarm main control units are similar to burglar alarms in the EMFs they give off. Fire alarm systems are sometimes triggered by

Smoke Detectors. Smoke detectors which are part of a central fire alarm system often have both temperature and infra-red detectors built in. These are quite safe and do not usually give off EMFs.

The most common type of smoke detectors are powered by a PP3 9 volt battery and do not give off any EMFs, however they do use a very low level radioactive source and should only be installed on ceilings and disposed of carefully if you renew them.

Treat **carbon monoxide detectors** in the same way as small battery-powered smoke detectors.

The **electricity meter** and main fuse is where the electricity supply from outside the house comes inside, ready for powering your electricity needs. This is where the meter reader takes his readings or where you insert your payment cards. The meter**, time switches, 'consumer units'** (or older **fuse boxes**) and the cables leading away give off quite high levels of electric and magnetic fields.

Modern all-electronic meters give off lower levels of magnetic fields compared with the older, 'spinning disc' electro-mechanical meters. If your electricity supplier wants to change your meter, you may want to ask which system they will be replacing it with, as some suppliers are experimenting with ones which give off microwaves similar to those from mobile phones. These latest design meters are intended to be remotely read without entering the house.

If your meter is outside the house, the house wall will give some protection from high electric fields. The high magnetic fields will *not* be reduced by the house wall. Do not place chairs next to the wall on the other side, especially if the chair is next to the telephone and intended to be used for long chats with friends and family.

If the meter is high up on the outside or inside wall, remember that the fields go upwards, perhaps into upstairs rooms, as well as sideways and downwards. Fields also go through to the other side of the wall, immediately behind the meter. This is especially important if you live in a flat or bungalow, with a bedroom the other side. Extra care must be taken if anyone is suffering from an acute or chronic immune-system deficiency, such as ME, other post viral conditions, cancers, people convalescing, and those having major medical treatments.

In flats, apartment or tenement blocks there is always a 'mains services riser' where electricity, gas, drains, etc., travel up through the building. Areas near the riser can have particularly high magnetic fields. The lower the floor you live on the higher the fields are likely to be, the highest being on the ground floor. We would always recommend measuring the EMFs if you live in such a situation.

The **consumer unit or fusebox** may be next to the electricity meter or away from it. It does not usually contain a transformer and so the magnetic fields created are just from the layout of the cables and the currents they are supplying. Wire fuses are just as good as circuit breakers, but the latter are more reliable.

Mechanical **time-switches** will contain a small motor but the fields from these do not extend for more than about half a metre.

Storage heaters may be your main form of heating, in the hall and / or elsewhere. Most heaters only draw on electricity through the night, when the electricity is off-peak and cheaper. Check with your electricity supplier if you are in doubt about what supply tariff you are on. They are full of high-density thermally absorbent material which can store the heat. During the day they gradually radiate the heat that they absorbed during the night, cooling down as they do so, until they once again switch on in the small hours of the morning and the cycle re-starts. During the daytime part of the cycle, the heaters give off heat, but no EMFs. At night, they can give off quite high levels of EMFs. Some electricity tariffs allow one or two extra short charging periods during the day when the heater will also be giving off high magnetic fields. On the ground floor of a house, there may not be anyone next to, or the other side of the wall from the heater at night; upstairs might be different. We will refer to storage heaters again when we extend the tour upstairs. If you are in a bungalow or flat, it is important to be aware of where beds are in relation to any of the storage heaters. Allow at least one metre between the heater and a bedhead.

Other types of heaters such as electric **convector heaters, oil filled radiators, electric radiant 'bar'** and **infrared heaters** give off magnetic fields close by. Be careful of chair and bed positions – half a metre away is usually adequate.

If you have **central heating**, your **boiler, pump and timer** might be in the hall. Remember that *all* forms of central heating have pumps and timers powered by electricity, even if the main fuel is oil, gas, or solid fuel. The **pumps** give off high magnetic fields, which, of course, travel through walls. Be careful about the position of chairs and beds where appropriate. **Hot air** central heating systems have a central fan which will give off significant levels of EMFs within about half a metre.

Central heating boilers do not generally give off any EMFs if they have a pilot light (flame) which burns continuously. Otherwise, they will give off a short burst when the electronic ignition fires.

If your **Central heating timer** is electromechanical and rotates then it will give off a lowish magnetic field that drops off quite quickly. **Hot water radiators** that are part of central heating systems shouldn't give off EMFs, but some do! The ONLY way to tell if you have a problem is to use a magnetic field meter and measure the EMF levels. These high fields are due to wiring faults which can be either inside *or outside(!)* your property and are dealt with as Net currents in Chapter 6.

Underfloor heating can either be by electric cables or hot water pipes. Hot water pipes are usually fine, though they can suffer from problems caused by the wiring faults mentioned in the previous paragraph. We do not like electric heating cables as they can cause EMF 'hotspots'. If you have this form of heating, we would advise you to carefully measure and map out the fields so that you and your family can avoid the areas where the EMFs are highest.

Some halls contain a **telephone**. A normal wired telephone is unlikely to be a problem. If you are considering changing your telephone, don't throw it away, keep it as a spare or return it to the manufacturer for recycling. You may have an **answerphone** attached. Answerphones are usually supplied with plug-mounted transformers, so take the usual precautions to do with **transformers**.

Health problems (headaches, skin tingling and heating, fatigue, concentration and memory loss, even tumours) have been associated with analogue and digital **cordless phones.** We recommend that you use an ordinary telephone for most of your calls and only use a cordless phone when you are away from your main phone (e.g. in the garden). Keep calls *short* on cordless phones. We do not recommend that children use them at all. In good signal reception areas, mobile phones can often emit less microwave power than digital cordless phones.

The main **base-unit** of digital cordless phones (DECT) emits pulses of microwaves, like the phone itself. Move away from the main base unit when you use the phone to avoid a double-whammy! The main base unit will emit microwaves every time the phone rings, but will stop if you then pick up the call on an ordinary wired (land-line or cable) telephone - but remember to replace the cordless phone on its stand to ensure the radiation is switched off. All the digital phone base units (including the charger units) give off high levels of low frequency fields and should not be put next to where you sit or sleep. The main unit will emit low frequency fields at all times it is plugged in to the mains even when the telephone is not in use.

Humidifier / de-humidifiers have electric motors and should be further away than normal, at least 1.2 metres away from chairs and beds. The water reservoir inside needs to be regularly cleaned and disinfected as the bacteria, fungi and moulds that can grow inside can produce runny noses, breathing problems and headaches.

Light switches and wiring can give off high levels of electric fields. A common cause of high magnetic fields are incorrectly wired **two-way** hall/landing **switches**. See Chapter 6 for more detail. Electric field levels rise considerably towards ceilings and this is almost always due to the way lighting wiring has been done since the 1950s. You can often trace where the wires go in the walls by following a line of high electric field, from the light switch upwards. When the wiring is in earthed metal conduit pipes (as originally was standard practice - and still is in public buildings) electric fields become almost non-existent. Electrical power **sockets** always give off electric fields. Sometimes there are high electric field levels all over walls, due to "leakage" and / or residual damp.

From the hall, we move into the sitting room. This includes any rooms in the house that are used extensively for leisure purposes. You may have more than one room that serves this purpose. Some equipment (e.g. computers, radio transmitters, typewriters etc.) will be discussed later as if they were in a separate room, an "office" as many people do use spare rooms, if available, for these activities. Some equipment e.g. hearing aids, wheelchairs, stairlifts etc. specifically for people who have special needs are discussed in Chapter 4.

Let us start with heating and cooling systems. Most heaters have been considered in the hall section earlier. However, **fan heaters** are very portable and likely to be used in rooms other than the hall. They have electric fan motors and heating elements and should be kept at least 1.2 metres away from beds and chairs.

Do you remember hot summers? If you do, or don't like the heat, or get the odd 'hot flush', you might have some cooling equipment such as **air conditioners**. Large systems are likely to be mounted on an external wall and usually have the main 'works' in a box outside the house. These consist of motors and pumps and can give off very high levels of magnetic fields. You need to keep 1.5 metres away from this equipment. If you have double glazing and you cannot open windows, poorly maintained air-conditioning systems may become clogged with dirt and pollutants. The polluted air is then re-circulated and increases the spread of airborne micro-organisms and bacteria, making you more vulnerable to sickness. This may be more of a problem in working environments.

For individuals, you might use a portable fan. These desk **fans** contain an electric motor which gives off quite high magnetic fields. Some only have a two-wire lead and are not 'earthed,' so they also tend to give off higher than usual electric fields. Keep the wire away from the person sitting near the fan, and preferably 'earth' the fan as well, see Chapter 6. **Ceiling fans** are not very common in houses in this country. They contain an electric motor which will give off quite high magnetic fields. You will not experience these in the room being cooled, but there will be a magnetic 'hotspot' immediately above, and extending outwards and upwards (depending on the strength of the motor) in the room above. Young children can play for long periods of time on the floor, so it is worth bearing this in mind, depending on whose bedroom may be above the fan. Shops and restaurants sometimes have them, which may be worth bearing in mind if you have a flat above such premises. You might remember to check playing and sleeping arrangements when you go abroad, where ceiling fans are more common.

Sitting rooms have a different range of systems of **lighting**. Usually there is a central light, which may hang down from the ceiling. Most normal incandescent lamps emit minimal EMFs other than heat and light, except from the flex. Most **fluorescent** lights give off higher electric and magnetic fields. Some high-efficiency, '**energy-saving**' **bulbs** (all fluorescent) give off VERY high localised magnetic fields. 'Electronic ballast' ones are better, but some of these give off radiofrequency radiation instead. Flicker and hum associated with older fluorescent lights, may be noticeable and trigger irritability, eyestrain and headaches.

You may have **standard lamps** and **table lamps** which can give off higher than usual electric fields as most only have a two-core mains lead - the leads themselves are the worst offenders and should be kept well away from your body. Any house in which children play regularly on the floor, should have appliance leads tied safely away, running along skirting boards wherever possible. This makes practical safety sense, it also protects them from high electric fields from the wires which are present even when the appliance's switch is off. The wire of a table lamp should lead away from the side of the base to the person sitting next to it.

Many people like to use spotlights to highlight a particular item of interest, or to create a well-defined localised pool of light. **Spotlights** are not normally a problem unless they are **halogen lights**. Halogen lights are fed by a low voltage transformer which gives off high magnetic fields. This transformer may be an integral part of the light fitting or separate. Wherever it is, you should sit at least one metre away from it. Some models emit levels of ultraviolet radiation towards your eyes when you are standing close by that can exceed international safety guidance.

Children, and those with skin cancer should be protected from high levels of UV radiation. In some instances high UV levels may react adversely with airborne pollutants, like tobacco smoke, resulting in photochemical smog. **Full-spectrum bulbs** do give out slightly higher levels of UV than standard bulbs but the more 'natural' light they emit is generally considered healthier to be in.

Most sitting rooms have at least one television set. Many houses have several sets. The general principles outlined here should be applied to all sets. We will discuss televisions in bedrooms again later, as it is important to ensure safe watching, especially with regard to children.

Colour **televisions** give off higher EMFs than black and white sets. Field levels vary from make-to-make - so unless you have measured the fields from your particular set and have got accurate information to guide you, always sit at least 1 metre away from the front of the screen. The age and size of the set is no guideline. Some new sets can be as bad as old sets; small screens can be as bad as big screens. Children should have a "no go" area, which is strictly adhered to. The back and side of the set also give off high fields - and remember that magnetic fields travel through walls. The backs of TV sets give off X-rays as well. One child we met had developed leukaemia, we believe possibly as a result of holding on to his TV set when learning to stand, and bouncing up and down to the music he heard on the set. The family were unaware of the need to keep him at a safe distance and were devastated by his illness.

Televisions also generate static electricity. That is why dusters can *always* pick up dust off a television screen. Use an antistatic cloth for best effect. A problem of this effect is that static electricity attracts anything that comes near it that is small enough. Some ongoing research from Bristol University shows that the dust attracted is a rich source of viruses, bacteria, and carcinogenic (cancer-inducing) particles. These can be floating in the air and are attracted to the TV screen, where they stick, rather than fall to the floor where they are vacuumed away. They may then be breathed in, or sucked off fingers that have been touching the screen. This is another reason for children to sit at a reasonable distance from a TV screen. The static effect persists (remember the dust?) for some time after the television has been switched off, so a "no-go" area as mentioned above is a good rule to insist on at all times.

Video recorders and **players** can also give off high fields if not 'earthed', which is a common situation.

Ensure that your TV is switched off using the main switch on the set. Switching it off by using some types of **remote control** means that your TV is on standby and continues to consume up to a quarter of the energy it uses when fully switched on. Most **remote control units** now use infra-red signals to transmit the control messages and these units do not produce concerning EMF levels.

EMFs from **digital TVs** are not much different in level from older analogue models.

Some TV screens are used as a monitor for **computer games,** e.g. Playstation, SEGA, SNES, etc.). Often neither the TV nor the game controller is connected to mains 'earth' and so the hand controllers can give off electric fields of several hundred volts per metre. The levels are unpredictable. It is very important to earth the equipment, see chapter 6.

The games units usually have a mains transformer, giving off high magnetic field levels, which plugs into a power socket. It is important to keep children away from them and to unplug the transformers when not in use. It is *very* important not to leave transformers plugged into the wall by children's beds as they leak quite high levels of magnetic fields all the time they are connected to the mains electricity supply.

As an alternative to broadcast entertainment, you might show a film of the last barbecue you had in the garden when Aunty Mabel came to visit, or the fabulous slides you found in the Greek islands of all the archaeological sites. To do this you will need a **film or slide projector**. These contain a motorised fan and solenoid which give off high fields up to about half a metre. Beyond this distance, they are not an EMF hazard.

Most sitting rooms have a **Music Centre, Hi-Fi unit**, an **audio-cassette** and/or **CD** player, with inbuilt or separate **loudspeakers**. None of these normally pose an EMF problem but the audio system should be earthed. Often the main amplifier has an earthing terminal on the back panel and this should be connected to mains earth. This is all that needs to be done. If the amplifier does not have an earth terminal, but instead has a three-core mains lead, then the earth will be connected internally. Portable equipment also used in bedrooms should be unplugged at night if within one metre of the bed. Cassette and CD players can contain a transformer which will continue to give off high fields if switched off at the appliance, but still switched on at the wall socket. This is especially important if you are unsure whether the system is earthed.

You may have a **radio** in the sitting room or elsewhere in the house. If it is a portable unit with a two-core mains lead, then this will give off electric and magnetic fields all the time it is connected to the mains. You should sit at least one metre away from it when listening and should always unplug it or switch it off at the wall after use.

Many people use **personal radios** and **stereo** systems either in the house or outside. Personal music systems (radio, CD and / or tape player, etc.) do not pose an EMF problem while being run on batteries. You may use **headphones** or encourage others to use them if one person's tastes in music are very different to those of other people in the same room! Be wary of the new cordless microwave headphone units. The headphones do not pose any danger, but we do not recommend sitting next to the base unit which is a microwave transmitter unit.

Home music makers may have a range of electric instruments. The most common are likely to be **electric guitars**, **keyboards** and the **amplifiers** that go with them. These latter may be used more in larger rooms, public halls, schools and colleges, etc. for very good reason! These are usually 'earthed' systems and do not pose an EMF hazard.

After all this loud music you may want to de-stress yourself watching the fish in an **aquarium**. The pumps that oxygenate most aquariums give off very high magnetic fields. Do not place chairs within about half a metre of the pumps. Aquarium heaters are not normally earthed and can leak electricity into the water causing the whole tank to give off suprisingly high electric fields.

You might have an **electric clock**. These are usually placed quite high on the wall, so are unlikely to be within a metre of where you sit. Battery-powered clocks do not give off high fields.

When you are getting ready for your night out (or in), you might wash and dry your hair. Drying and/or styling your hair can involve different types of equipment. **Hair curlers** that are preheated and put in your hair, using the retained heat to dry it and give it the shape you want are all right. The heating units, which are heated directly by electricity, will give off significant EMF levels. When you have removed the curlers, it is a good idea to switch the heating unit off at the wall. If you might want to re-heat the curlers, sit away from the heating unit whilst it is still working. **Curling tongs** are a self-contained, heated unit. It will give off quite high fields, depending on the heat setting. The metal construction will distort the magnetic field, which can increase the effects. We do not recommend their use at all, but especially not in the evening.

Hand-held **hairdryers** use high currents to produce heat. The motor gives off very high fields near the handle, dropping only a little at normal drying distances (6 to 18 inches). The fields are higher when it is on a "high heat" setting than when it is on a "low heat" setting. The fact that a hairdryer is only used for a few minutes each time, is not as important as the fact that the user is exposed to *very high fields indeed* while it *is* working. Metal hair clips can make the effect worse.

We recommend that no hair dryers should be used after 7.00 p.m. at the very latest. High magnetic fields near the head in the evening are known to interfere with the production of melatonin by the pineal gland (see Chapter 1). It is best to wash your hair in the morning, or at a time when you can allow it to dry naturally, whenever possible. **Hood hairdryers** have a very high field. There is usually more than one heat setting; the fields will be higher as the heat is greater. Sitting still under the hood regularly may have an adverse effect. Any metal securing curlers, or metal parts used in the curler construction etc. will increase the harmful effect. Wall mounted hair dryer units, that use a simple air pipe to take the warm air to the head are a good idea.

So you're now back home after a heavy day at work, or a good night out. How about a **foot spa**? Foot spas have a motorised pump and usually an electric heater - and will generate EMFs. The benefits will probably outweigh the disadvantages, as your feet are not as sensitive as other parts of your body to the effects of EMFs.

In the kitchen, a veritable Aladdin's cave of electrical treasures awaits us. If you are concerned about potential adverse health effects from electrical appliances, it may be worth reviewing the equipment you have, deciding whether you actually need it, and where it should be located.

The primary purpose of kitchens is usually preparing and cooking food. Sometimes it also includes the dining area.

We make a start with cooking facilities. These can come in all sorts of combinations these days, from the more traditional hot plates, grill, and oven combination cooker, to fan assisted ovens, double ovens, toaster ovens; and separate hobs, including those with ceramic, halogen and magnetic induction plates.

The traditional electric **cooker** gives off high magnetic fields when it is operating. These can be very high close to. In a small kitchen, there may not be much room when food is actually being cooked to keep very far away. If this is the case, it is a good idea to prepare the uncooked food first and then perhaps move to a different room when the food is cooking, only going in to check on progress briefly. Pregnant women should certainly do this, as the highest field levels from the oven can be in the area of the growing unborn child, depending on the dimensions of the cooker and the mother's own height. The bigger the kitchen, the easier it is to stay doing other things whilst the cooker is working.

Children should not play in front of the cooker, especially the oven, while it is on. This is unlikely because of safety risks from pans on the hot plates etc., but it is worth while making sure that their normal playing area is at least a metre away from the front of the cooker.

The average time spent cooking is about one hour a day, apparently, according to research. This is almost certain to vary according to the time of year. If you spend longer than this it is worthwhile taking especial care. All electrical **fan assisted ovens, double ovens, toaster ovens, grills, time switches,** etc. give off significant magnetic fields. Keep the usual distance away whilst they are working.

You might be using a separate **hob** at the same time as the oven is on elsewhere in the kitchen. Pregnant women, especially, are not advised to stand in front of it for longer than necessary. Perhaps it's a good time to develop the cooking skills of other members of the family! How about eating out? Pregnant professional cooks may want to consider their work environments, making any possible necessary changes. **Ceramic** and **halogen hobs** generate similar levels of magnetic fields as conventional open-ring electric hobs.

Hobs with **magnetic induction plates** work on a different heating principle. VERY strong EMFs are deliberately generated by the cooker to make currents flow in the pans themselves, which causes them to heat up. The top of the cooker stays relatively cool and is only heated by contact with the hot pan. As high EMFs are generated on purpose, we cannot recommend this way of cooking. As physical cells are changed by high EMFs, it is uncertain what effect this might have on the food, especially if eaten by people with immune system problems. Some magnetic induction plates use mains frequency fields and some use low radio frequency signals which can induce currents in the pan (and people standing nearby!) more easily.

Slow cookers usually use very low power and do not pose a significant EMF hazard.

Many cookers have a **hood** above them extracting the cooking fumes. The fields from electric hood motors are high up to about half a metre away. You are not likely to spend much time standing in front of it, but it may be a good idea to limit the time when it is dark, as the high fields generated will be at about head height and this can affect the production of melatonin (the body's detoxifier), for the following night-time period. The same will apply to other **extractor fans**. Motors generate high EMFs and if the fan is close to your head, keep the time you spend nearer than about a metre to it to a minimum when it is on.

Most families contain at least one chip-addict. A **deep-fat fryer** will give off high EMFs as the oil is heated. For safety reasons you should not leave the fryer while it is working. Perhaps this is another reason for reducing chip consumption as well as nutritional reasons. Used infrequently, it shouldn't be a problem. If the work surface on which it is placed is at a critical height, due to the cook's pregnancy or a tendency to prostate cancer in the family, take extra care.

If your local electricity company has measured the fields inside your house, they will almost certainly measure your **microwave oven** to show you what high fields you live with. Microwave ovens generate two types of radiation; low frequency radiation from the strong power transformer that can give off up to 30,000 nT at 15 cm and 2,000 nT at 1 metre; they also use microwave (high frequency) radiation to cook the food. This radiation can leak out through the door glass and from around the door seals. Since microwave emissions can change with normal use, ovens should be checked regularly, preferably annually, to pick up any microwave leakage. See Chapter 8 for details of the Microlarm detector.

Even when the oven is working correctly, the microwave levels within the kitchen are likely to be significantly higher than those from any nearby cellular phone base-stations. Despite the fact that most microwave ovens are used for only short periods of time, as the fields are so high it is important to take proper safety precautions.

We recommend that *nobody* stands nearer than 1 metre from the oven when it is on. If the kitchen is small, it is a good idea to encourage children to stay out of the kitchen whilst the microwave oven is on. *On no account* should they stand in front of it to watch the food cooking. This can frequently happen when children are hungry, or fascinated by some of the changes which become visible as the food cooks. This also applies to anyone whose immune system is not working well.

All microwave oven manufacturers recommend you leave food to stand for 2-3 minutes after cooking (for reasons of taste) and they are often ignored. **It is important to wait!** Do not just warm food up. Heat thoroughly, and leave to stand for 2-3 minutes before eating or drinking. This is to allow for re-absorption of free radicals created in the heating process. Free radicals are known to have carcinogenic properties.

In America, it was found that a third of ovens tested did not heat mashed potato up enough to destroy bacteria. With the increase in concern about salmonella and listeria, we suggest you use other forms of cooking for most of yours and your family's meals.

Babies' bodies and cell structures are much more vulnerable even than older children's. Baby bottles should ***not*** be heated to body temperature and immediately given to babies. We do not recommend a microwave oven for the cooking or heating up of **any** baby foods.

Electric **bottle warmers** for baby bottles are fine and only give off low levels of EMFs, although some only have a two-wire connection and so give off AC electric fields.

Most people boil water in an **electric kettle.** Both the older style ones and the more modern jug-type create high EMFs. Keep the heating kettle at a reasonable distance. Heating water using electricity can change its molecular structure. Some people react badly to this change. If *you* do, to neutralise this effect, stand the mug, cup or glass on a strong magnet while you pour the water into it.

Sandwich makers are used briefly. Switch off at the wall immediately when finished. For many models this is the only option to being fully on, as they do not have an off switch on the machine. Similar comments apply to **toasters.**

Food processors, mixers and **blenders** all contain motors. They give off high EMFs close to which drop away rapidly. Short periods of use should be no problem. Give some thought as to how many electric appliances giving off high fields at work-top height you expose yourself to during pregnancy. Perhaps limiting the number of electrically powered machines you use during the day is worth considering.

The same comments are basically true for **coffee grinders** and **coffee makers**. You might choose to change from an electric coffee maker to a cafetière method, which does not use electricity. I guess hand-grinding beans wouldn't be most people's choice. Why not give up coffee, it's bad for your stress levels anyway?

Do you really need an **electric can opener**? Medical conditions such as arthritis may justify their use. Otherwise, we recommend a mechanical one. The same for **electric knives**. Reducing the number of electric gadgets you use reduces your cumulative exposure to EMFs.

When your food is cooked, it is sometimes useful to keep it warm while the conversation flows at the dinner table. **Hostess trolleys** can be used to transport the hot food and plates to the dining room and to keep the food warm while you eat. They use electric warming elements which do not use much power, so EMF hazards are minimal. There are non-electrical alternatives which might be worth thinking about.

All this cooking results in dirty dishes. Modern **dishwashers** use less water (about 20 litres) for a family of four, than washing dishes by hand (about 40 litres). They are probably more hygienic, as the dishes do not need drying, and most dishtowels harbour germs however well looked after. However, a lot of energy is used in the manufacture of the machines; they use a lot of energy to heat the water and to dry the dishes. The decision whether to use a dishwasher is more complex than just about EMFs. If your dishwasher is on an outside wall ensure good insulation as it can be very energy consuming in this position. Always have a full load. EMFs can be high when the machine is operating. This is important to bear in mind especially if small children are likely to play in the kitchen while it is working. The only way to be sure where the 'safe' field level is, is to measure the fields. Try using a timer device so that you use night-time off-peak electricity, keeping EMF exposure to a minimum.

The highest fields from a **freezer** or a **fridge** are from the motor. Make sure you know where the motor is and keep a reasonable distance. A full freezer is more efficient, and a chest freezer is more efficient than an upright one. To reduce EMF exposure and improve energy efficiency, site a chest freezer in an unheated garage. Fridges are often put close to cookers when kitchens are small. This means that the motor has to work hard to keep the inside temperature down. This leads to higher EMFs and reduced energy efficiency, not to mention higher running costs. A well-stocked fridge uses less power than a poorly-stocked one, since more energy is needed to cool empty space. Keep the freezer compartment of your fridge clear of ice. The same thing applies to **fridge / freezers**.

By the sink, you may have a **water heater**. With central heating, when the system heats the water all year round they are less common. You may have one for supplemental heating for when the main system is switched off. The heater will give off highish EMFs similar to an electric kettle. They are usually positioned some way away from the body, but at head height. Be aware of your exposure time in the evenings when it is dark and your pineal gland is susceptible to being 'switched off'.

The motor powering a kitchen **waste disposal unit** will be in the space underneath the sink. It is likely to have quite a high-powered motor, which will give off high EMFs when in operation. Take care to minimise exposure. Build a compost heap instead and let the worms do the work for you. The more organic waste that is put into the waste water system, the more expensive it is to re-purify the water at sewage works. Then we all pay higher water rates to cover the increased cost.

If you live in a hard water area, you may have bought an in-line **water softener.** Some water softeners use magnetism to change the molecular structure of the impurities in the water which create the scale that blocks pipes and causes 'scum' in the washing. Some scientists believe that these molecular structure changes can cause biological reactions and long-term health problems if you drink the water. If you want to soften the water for the sake of pipes and equipment that fails if scale builds up, then try to keep drinking water separate from the water softening system. The water can be softened to some extent by using a jug-type **water filter**, which filters out many of the harmful minerals. Or you might use bottled water, especially for people with compromised immune systems. Many bottled waters are quite contaminated with microbes and bacteria, which does not prevent their being sold quite legally, so do your research. Inline water filters requiring pumps may have subtle molecular effects on drinking water which may be undesirable.

We have visited houses that have had their household **water supply** affected by sources of electricity outside the house. Sometimes the way that electricity substations are interconnected generate 'net' currents (for more details see Chapter 3). When electricity cables and mains water pipes share the same trenches in the street distribution system, the water supply pipe can enter a house carrying an EMF 'charge'. As a result, current then flows around the house through the water pipes feeding central heating radiators, bathroom showers, etc., causing high levels of magnetic field. Remedial action is necessary.

If you live in a high-risk area for radon, such as the South West of England, this radioactive gas, formed by the decay of uranium, is likely to be absorbed by your water supply. Get your radon levels checked and take remedial action if necessary.

Some houses have a separate utility room. We have also included some items of electrical equipment in this section that didn't seem to belong anywhere else.

Washing machines are usually in the kitchen or a separate utility room. If your machine is in the kitchen, the problems caused by high EMFs when the machine is working are more obvious than if it is in a room that you use less often or for less time. Close to they give off high fields of several microtesla ($1\mu T$ = 1,000nT). Washing machines are often pushed under work surfaces. We recommend you do not work close by these appliances or let children play in front of them, whilst they are in operation. Ideally, install a timer, so the machine can run at night on cheaper-rate electricity, when no-one is around.

Spinners extract excess water from hand-washed material, before drying. The motor gives off high EMFs. Some spinners are used on the floor, and are fine. The smaller units which are put on draining boards, will give off lower fields as they will probably have a less powerful motor, but the fields will radiate potentially more vital body areas.

Once the clothes are washed, they then need to be dried. Drying clothes in wet winter weather can often be a problem. We turn to all sorts of electrical appliances to help resolve this problem.

A combined **washer/dryer** is similar to the two separate appliances for generating power frequency magnetic field levels. **Tumble dryer** motors give off similar high fields to washing machines. Keep yourself and children at a reasonable distance. Keep the filter clean to improve efficiency. A tumble dryer generally costs more to run than a washing machine, so use when necessary only. Separate **clothes dryers** which have an airer unit attached to a floor-based heater give off quite a high magnetic field. Do not let children play near, especially in the winter when the heat may be attractive to them. As the base unit is usually metal, you are unlikely to allow them to get too near for other safety reasons.

Electric **irons** have very low fields and are not a problem, though pregnant women should try to keep the iron at least 30 cm from their body. Try getting someone else to do the ironing for you! **Trouser presses** and **electric mangles** give off low EMFs and are not a problem over half a metre away.

Electric **sewing machine** motors give off high magnetic fields. Some machines with two-core mains cables give off high electric fields. Statistically significant increases in Alzheimer's disease have been detected in machinists using industrial machines. Be aware of where the motor is, and if you are in a susceptible group, change to a mechanically-driven machine for lengthy use.

Floor polishers have motors which give off high fields. Try to keep your feet at least half a metre away when they are in use.

The type of **vacuum cleaner** that runs over the floor, with an attached suction hose is better than an upright cleaner, as the motor and wires are further away from you. Hand-held cleaners, such as those used to vacuum furniture or cars, produce high fields next to your body.

Most **sun beds** give off high electric and magnetic fields as well as possibly dangerous levels of ultra-violet radiation. Many can give off five times as much UVA as would be expected from bright sunlight at the equator. They increase the risk of skin cancer, especially in fair-skinned people. **Sun lamps** are OK for general EMFs but the ultra-violet comments applied to sunbeds also apply here. Ultra-violet is a form of non-ionising radiation that we know causes skin cancers.

Exercise machines are generally not a problem. Remember that motors (such as those used to power treadmills etc.) give off high magnetic fields close to. Maybe the exercise is more beneficial than the small level of potential risk.

In this part we have put equipment that may be elsewhere in your house, or you may not have at all. It includes what might be used by some people working from home. The most common appliance will be the **computer**. Most modern computers give off quite low levels of fields. As always, to minimise EMF exposure try to keep the computer, especially the display, as far away from your body as is practical.

There have been extensive investigations, into the potential hazards of **computer display monitors** sometimes known as **VDUs**

(Visual Display Unit). Most of this research was done in the USA, as this is where the IT revolution began. Old cathode ray tube (CRT) type screens can give off high electromagnetic fields and x-rays. These have been associated with miscarriages and birth defects in women who have used VDUs at work. If you are concerned about VDUs we recommend the book produced by the London Hazards Centre listed in Chapter 8. The vast majority of VDU operators in the US are women and the incidence of female breast cancer has been rising steadily along with VDU use. Other less severe problems sometimes associated with VDUs are high levels of stress, headaches, anxiety, fatigue, nausea, depression, dizziness, irritability, skin redness or rashes, and eye strain.

Newer, low radiation, computer screens complying with the Swedish **MPRII** guidelines give off far lower ELF (Extremely Low Frequency) fields. The newer **TCO-95** guideline levels are even lower. It is worth checking whether your monitor complies with these standards, especially if it is given to you second-hand, and may predate them. This can occasionally be a problem for schools having well-meaning, but uninformed benefactors. There will be a label on the rear of the monitor showing any standards that it meets. Always sit at least an arm's length from the front of the screen.

All traditional Cathode Ray Tube VDUs give off higher fields at the back and sides. Nobody should sit less than 1 metre from the rear of a VDU, at home, or in the office. It is worth remembering that magnetic fields travel through walls, so watch the use of the room next door. Smaller VDU's are not necessarily better, either, because the field's strength depends more on the internal design than on the screen size. Shields placed in front of a VDU's screen do not block magnetic fields. Most so-called shields just remove reflections from windows and room lights and do nothing to reduce EMFs.

Modern 'TFT' flat screen monitors give off virtually no EMFs at all. They are similar to the screens used in the best lap-top computers. They do, at present, cost over double the price of a conventional monitor.

Screen savers designed to blank out the screen after a short period of inactivity are useful to prevent "burn in" or damage to the VDU's phosphor coating from constant use, but even if the image is dark, the components which generate EMF emissions are still active. Similarly, dimming the display will do nothing to reduce the fields.

When you buy a new computer monitor, it is a good idea to leave it switched on in an unused well-ventilated room for about two weeks. The casing contains fire-retardant chemicals that are given off when the computer is working. These can produce quite toxic side-effects in people who use them and at worst could provoke electrical sensitivity.

You should ideally take a 15 minute break every hour when using a VDU. If this is not possible, at least 5 minutes, leaving the desk area. If the image on your monitor is unstable, flickers or wobbles, it is almost certainly in magnetic fields which are far too high for you to work in. Under European and UK legislation, it is now illegal to have to work with an unstable monitor image (Display Screen Equipment Regulations).

Lap Top Computers (with LCD or TFT screens) generally give off very low EMFs. However, when run from mains adapters they can give off VERY high electric fields next to the keyboard and display. This can cause sensitive people severe problems. The answer is to charge them up away from where you sit, and then run them off their internal re-charged batteries, or see the details in Chapter 6 about earthing such two-wire appliances when in use.

Anglepoise lamps are often used to give focused light at desks. Metal framed lamps can give off very high electric fields due to the practice of wiring lights with two-core flex. This can obviously cause a problem if you spend a lot of time (working from home, or conscientiously doing homework, etc.) with your head close to the lamp. Always use three core flex and connect the earth wire to the metal frame (Chapter 6).

Pagers and **beepers** generally do not give off harmful EMFs, although 'advanced' pagers can transmit microwave signals. These are not very common and we do not know if they are available in the UK.

Electric **pencil sharpeners** have motors which do give off high EMFs but are not usually a hazard as they are only used occasionally for short periods. They add to your overall EMF exposure, so consider whether they are really necessary, especially if you are pregnant.

Photocopiers can give off very high magnetic fields close to the motor. Find out where the motor is situated in the photocopier and stand back at least 50 cm. while it is copying. Always ventilate the room well as the ozone given off by the copier is affected by the surrounding electric fields. Toner powder is toxic when inhaled and is attracted to static electricity, such as you will find on the photocopier plate where the paper to be copied is placed, and elsewhere in the machine. Great care should be taken when changing the toner cartridge.

Laser **printers** give off ozone, and also use toner (see photocopiers). Unless you really need the slightly better quality of a laser printer, a good quality inkjet or squirtjet printer is much more economical (on consumables) and ecological.

Most **Scanners** give off negligible fields, although some have separate mains transformers, which give off high magnetic fields.

Electric **typewriters** are usually MUCH worse than computers for EMFs. If you have to use one, **switch it off at the socket** when you are not actually typing. The ones we have measured give off very high magnetic fields (because of cheaply constructed internal transformers) and some, with only two-wire mains leads, give off high electric fields at the keyboard. Be very wary about using one at all if you are pregnant.

Faxes give off similar fields to electric typewriters.

Amateur (Ham) radio transmitters can emit very high levels of radiofrequency and microwave radiation and should be relegated to a shed at the bottom of the garden, and not installed in the house. Most of the radiation is associated with the aerials and can extend for a considerable distance around them. Amateur UHF Moon-Bounce transmitters use a highly focused aerial array with extremely high power in the main beam. These arrays should be kept away from children's play areas and neighbouring houses.

Time to go upstairs.

Let us remind ourselves of storage heaters that might be on the landing, heating the first floor. At night, they give off high magnetic fields, which travel through walls. Be very careful about what is the other side, especially children's beds.

We often find the airing cupboard on the landing, containing the immersion heater, and frequently timing devices. The **immersion heater** and its wiring will give off high magnetic fields. Bedheads should be at least 1 metre away from the immersion heater cupboard wall.

Cleanliness being next to Godliness, we will follow divine footsteps to the bathroom.

The water-heater element used in **electric showers** is very powerful and gives off several microtesla 30 cm away. It is wise not to stand too close to the control unit especially in the evening due to the pineal gland effect (see Chapter 1).

If you live in a high-risk area for radon, such as the South West of England, this radioactive gas, formed by the decay of uranium, can enter your water supply. It is then dispersed and inhaled in the form of hot steam from the shower or bath.

An **electric shaver** which plugs into the wall produces an extremely high electric field half an inch away from the cutting edge. The data on short-term exposure to high-strength fields is incomplete, and the use of non-electric razors will eliminate all EMF risks. The magnetic fields, being close to the brain, could influence production of melatonin, especially if the razor is used in the evening. We recommend using rechargeable battery shavers which are easily obtainable. Battery-powered shavers still give off quite high magnetic fields from the motor, but we do not believe they present a hazard for the short periods they are in use.

The batteries powering an **electric toothbrush** are charged up on a separate unit. This is unlikely to be kept in a problem place.

There are not many houses which have **jacuzzis.** If your house does, some jacuzzis have pumps and motors built in to the base which will result in your being exposed to high EMF exposure. We do not believe that short-term use in a hotel is a problem, but if the jacuzzi is in your house, then we recommend that the pumps and motors are at least half a metre away from the bath.

Other equipment that might be in bathrooms will have been dealt with elsewhere.

To bedrooms... to sleep, perchance to dream.... and the best sleepers are babies; or most of them anyway.

There are items in baby's and children's rooms that are less likely to be in other bedrooms.

The best type of **baby alarms** are the battery-operated, wire connected, alarms which give off virtually zero fields. Alarms plugged into the mains give off high fields and should be at least 1 metre away from the baby's bedhead. The walk-about 'freedom' alarms radiate radio-frequency energy next to the child in order to communicate with the parents' listening unit. We cannot recommend this type of system.

Nightlights enable adults and children to see each other and children to see their surroundings, if they do not like to sleep in the dark. It is preferable that everybody sleeps in dark conditions if achievable, because these are the conditions in which the pineal gland best produces melatonin, the body's natural anti-cancer hormone. If necessary, have a low-wattage bulb, in a unit well away from the child's bed, ensuring the wires, which give off electric fields even when the bulb is off at the switch, are well away from the bed. Candle nightlights are, of course, fine with normal precautions taken with naked flames.

Many **dimmer switches** and their associated wiring tend to give off radiofrequency noise. Most give off quite high electromagnetic fields up to a few inches from the light switch and wires (even when wires are embedded in the wall, unless they are in metal conduit). Care needs to be taken with regard to siting bunk beds, for instance, to ensure adequate distance between the switch and the head of a child.

The construction of some beds give more EMF problems than others. **Beds** with metal frames and bedsprings can become magnetised due to domestic wiring and electrical appliances in the bedroom, causing restlessness and insomnia. These bedframes can be de-gaussed, thus removing the fields. This is difficult to do and there are very few places in Britain where it can be done. If you believe this is the cause of your problem, find an alternative bed-base and unsprung mattress, preferably with natural materials. Many futons achieve these standards, but may take some getting used to as they can be much firmer than sprung mattresses. Always keep electrical appliances of any sort at least 1 metre away from bedheads. Switch off at the wall, or unplug any appliances (e.g. bedside lights, electric blankets) that are closer than this, after use. **Do not have transformers plugged in next to a bedhead.** This can easily happen in children's rooms. Wherever possible, do not run electric wires behind the bed, even along the skirting board. You could put them under the carpet and put earthed aluminium foil over the top (see Appendix 2). Use screened cable in the wall, or metal conduit to reduce EMFs as near as possible to zero.

Water beds can give high electric and magnetic fields from the water heaters. It is inadvisable to sleep on this type of bed with the heater on through the night. Waterbeds should be warmed during the day, but unplugged before going to bed. However, an unheated water bed can get quite chilly, so you may need a thick mattress pad or quilt to stay warm.

It is not a good idea to use electrically-powered **heating pads** for chronic problems. You should replace them with hot water bottles.

Electric blankets create a magnetic field that penetrates about 6 or 7 inches into the body. Some firms sell "low-magnetic field" models, or blankets using DC electricity. Although these models reduce or eliminate magnetic fields, the blanket may still produce electric fields. The hot plastic coated wires release chemical fumes, which are themselves toxic.

Electric blankets can cause cramp. The rate of miscarriage has been found to be higher in women who use electric blankets. The most critical exposure time is the first three months of pregnancy. In one study, the children of women who used electric blankets early in pregnancy were four times as likely to develop cancer. Two studies showed that children who had used electric blankets were up to five times more likely to develop leukaemia, the commonest form of childhood cancer.

Electric overblankets which are designed to be left on overnight, are usually run from a low voltage transformer. Both the transformer and blanket give off even higher magnetic fields than underblankets. We recommend that you do not use such a blanket if you are concerned about EMFs.

Underblankets and overblankets should <u>always</u> be switched off before getting into bed. Unless you have 3-core screened cable attached to the blanket, it should be switched off at the wall (otherwise the wire will still give off electric fields between the socket and the blanket switch). This is one place where a 'Demand Switch' (details can be found towards the end of this Chapter) can be useful. A tufted lambs' wool underblanket, is a natural, safe way of keeping warm.

Bedhead lights and **bedside lights** give off high electric and magnetic fields. Most light cabling is two-core and so the wire still gives off electric fields even if the light is switched off using the light-switch. It is important to switch them off at the socket on the wall to prevent this. We recommend using screened mains cable for bedside lights, which earths the lamps. Be careful of where the wires go in relation to the bed. Some beds have wires running along the wall behind the bed, giving off high electric fields near the person's head throughout the night. Cables in the walls can also give off high magnetic fields. This is remedied by using metal conduit to contain the cabling. If you are unsure of the levels of field behind your bed, it can be advisable to move the bed six inches away from the wall. If you have a poor immune system or a serious illness, it is advisable to measure the fields and take appropriate remedial action if necessary. Lights give off high magnetic fields all the time they are switched on. It is a good idea to move them as far away from your head at night as is practical.

Televisions should always be **at least** four feet away from the pillow area. It is particularly important to earth TVs in bedrooms, because of the high electric fields. Keep the light levels down at night due to the pineal gland effect. Battery-operated **remote controls** are quite safe.

Children's bedrooms can resemble mini-laboratories with all the electric and electronic gadgetry they often like to have. The important things to be aware of are:

- Keep all electrical appliances at least four feet away from the bed.
- Switch everything off at the wall and preferably unplug them at night.
- Transformers are a special hazard and should never be plugged in near a bed.
- Do not keep anything electric, especially mains-powered tape and CD players on a shelf above the bed without unplugging them at the wall. Be wary of headphones (see sitting room section, or Chapter 5).
- When your children are unwell, limit the time they spend in front of a computer screen, especially a lap-top computer, to minimise the effect on their depleted immune system. It may be an idea to reduce the amount of microwaved food they eat at this time, unless it is a specific part of their treatment regime.

Clock radios, while very useful to wake you up with whatever may be your choice of early morning patter or music, should be kept at least four feet away from the nearest head, as they will be giving off high fields throughout the night. Older electro-mechanical clocks are worse than newer, electronic digital ones. If this is not possible, perhaps replacing it with a wind-up alarm may be a good idea. Then you can get up to switch on a radio; good for waking you up thoroughly.

Some people cannot cope with early morning radio without an early morning cup of tea - very wise, too! Remember the benefits of early morning exercise and put your **tea-making machine** at least four feet from the head of your bed, or go to the kitchen. A tea-maker does give off high fields when it is doing a brew-up, so it is important to keep some distance away.

The next two items are hardly electrical appliances, but we thought it was important to mention them.

Underwired bras can act as 'antennas' re-radiating external EMFs, including microwave frequencies, into the body. With the increase in rate of breast cancer and the genetic susceptibility that some women have to developing breast cancer, we cannot recommend the wearing of underwired bras.

All **wristwatches** with batteries give off significant magnetic pulses every time the mechanism is activated (possibly several times a second). It is unclear what effect that may have.

We have completed the tour of the inside of a generalised house. We hope that has given you an idea of what to look for and what to do.

The next brief section of this chapter is to answer some of the more general questions we have been asked about electricity in the home.

What are **demand switches?** and when would they be useful?

A demand switch automatically isolates **some** or **all** of the electrical circuits in the home, switching off the mains supply voltage once it is no longer needed. It then monitors the circuit using a very low voltage and re-applies the full mains voltage when you switch something on.

Downstairs circuits usually have equipment such as fridges and freezers on the circuit and therefore should not be switched off overnight. As discussed in the sections above, some machines such as dishwashers and washing machines can be used at off-peak times, reducing EMFs in the room when you are there and increasing energy efficiency. You will want to leave these on overnight powered circuits. Upstairs power circuits may be suitable for demand switches. Lighting circuits produce most of the electric fields in a house and are ideal candidates for a demand switch. Any lights left on all night for safety reasons will need to be fed from a separate circuit. Demand switches should be installed by qualified electricians. Currently demand switches are imported, largely from Germany. We are hoping to develop a British-made source. For more details, contact Powerwatch, the address and phone number are in Chapter 8.

Why do **electric light bulbs 'fail'** frequently?

If it is only light bulbs, check whether another make will give you more reliability. We bought a cheap lot at one point, and found they were failing after a very short time. We wrote it down to experience and paid more for the next lot, which lasted much longer. So much for economy! Most bulbs are only designed for 1000 hours continuous use and last for a shorter total time when switched on and off. Some are 'double life' and are guaranteed to last for 2000 hours. The best bulbs have 'coiled-coil' filaments which are less easily damaged by being switched on and off.

Most normal shaped bulbs are designed to be used with the globe part hanging downwards. If they are used in wall-light fittings with the connection end downwards (apparently "upside down") then they do not generally last as long.

See also the comment on supply voltage, below.

Why does **electrical equipment 'fail'** frequently?

If <u>one</u> item of electrical equipment <u>only</u> keeps giving problems, that item may be faulty.

If electric light bulbs and other electrical appliances are failing frequently, it is likely that your **supply voltage** is too high. This should be checked by a qualified electrician. For many years the UK supply voltage has been a nominal 240 volts a.c. (251 volts maximum). This has now been officially changed to 230 volts and many bulb suppliers may be changing their bulbs to give the same brightness at 230 volts. None of the electricity companies have announced (as at September 1999), when they are going to start to change their distribution systems over to the lower voltage. It is still legal to be supplied with a voltage of about 251 volts. Until the systems change to the lower voltage, light bulbs and other simple appliances may last for less time!

Measure your **supply voltage**. If it measures more than 245 volts, then complain to your electricity supplier and ask them to lower it. If your bulbs flicker frequently, you should ask your Regional Electricity Company to monitor the quality of your electricity supply.

Why does **electronic equipment** turn itself on & off?

If this is happening frequently, check that there is not a loose connection in the plug or socket and that the plug fuse is not loose. Hold the item and shake it (carefully!) to see if it has an internal loose connection, in which case you need to take it to an electrical repair shop. If nothing seems to be the problem with the equipment itself, there may be a source of radio frequency interference nearby. Try the item in another part of the house - preferably near ground level, and see if the problem persists. It is unlikely that equipment bought after 1995, and which has 'CE' marked on it, will be susceptible to anything other than a mobile phone being used within about three metres of it. All equipment now has to be certified not to malfunction below three volts per metre of RF and microwave energy. Mobile phones and microwave ovens can give off far more than this within about three metres. If you know of a radio amateur nearby, we suggest you contact the person and ask for their advice, as the problem may be due to their equipment. In any case, they will have learned about radio frequency interference (RFI) in order to obtain their licence. If you need further advice, we suggest you call our 0897 100 800 helpline to speak to Alasdair Philips.

Are **homoeopathic remedies** affected by electric or magnetic fields?

Homoeopathic remedies come in either tablet or liquid form. They are a product of water which is magnetically remembering the resonance frequencies of the original substance used to produce the remedy. The potency (effectiveness) of the remedy is made completely ineffective as a medicine if they are placed, even for a short time, next to a source of magnetic fields. This source could be a transformer, a television or radio loudspeaker or even a strong permanent magnet. They should be kept away from steel cabinets in case these are magnetised. Be aware of what material your bathroom cabinet is made from. Often car tyres are magnetised, due to the steel content. Do not place remedies above the wheel arches in a car.

CHAPTER THREE
AROUND AND ABOUT

Around your Home

Having toured the inside of your home, we now go outside to look at EMF sources, firstly attached to the house. **Satellite dishes and receivers** can give off high electric fields if the TV system or satellite decoder is not 'earthed' to the mains electricity safety earth. Most TVs, video recorders and satellite systems are not earthed when you buy them, as they only have two-wire mains leads. Walls will give some protection from the electric fields; windows are less effective at screening them. It is important that these systems are earthed (see Chapter 6).

Digital TV receptors for both satellite and terrestrial signals can be thought of in exactly the same way as satellite dishes and receivers. There is only a subtle difference in the way the information is coded into the signal. TV reception signals are very small indeed and are believed to have no biological effect. Some questions have been raised about the safety of living near large and powerful TV transmitting masts. You will find more information about these towards the end of this Chapter.

Many houses have some form of **security system** to detect unwanted intruders. Most intruder sensors should not cause EMF hazards outside your home. You should know how to switch off microwave sensors, for when you want to be in the garden or in other areas the sensors cover. If you do not know how, contact the installer and find out how this can be done.

Solar heating systems, to heat houses, are being promoted as they are based on a renewable source of energy, an alternative to fossil fuel. The system itself will not be an EMF hazard, except for the electric pump used to pump the water around. This could be outside or inside the house. Keep chairs, beds, etc. on the other side of the wall, at least one metre away from the pump.

The Garden & Workshop

Next, we have equipment used, or kept, in the garden. The most likely will be **electric lawn mowers** and **power tools** (drills, hedge trimmers, strimmers, sanders, etc.). All electric power tools give off

EMFs; those with motors close to your body (e.g. electric drills and hedgecutters) will give you high magnetic and electric field exposure while in use. There is nothing you can do about this and short term occasional exposure should not cause any EMF related problems, unless you are particularly sensitive. The motors of some tools and lawn mowers are further away from your body when in use and so the fields your body is exposed to are lower. The evidence seems to show that occupational exposure when you are moving about is less of a risk than prolonged exposure when you are stationary (i.e. in a chair or bed).

Soldering irons which plug directly into the mains electricity are unlikely to be a problem. Many modern soldering irons run from a low-voltage transformer / controller unit which does give off high magnetic fields and should be situated conveniently at arm's length from your working position.

When your lawn and garden are looking good, it may be time to invite neighbours, friends and family for a barbecue.

Barbecues are rarely electrical and, anyway, are only used for short periods and so will not pose a problem. Should you decide to record the event for future viewing, your **camcorder** motor gives off high fields, but is well shielded, so the person doing the filming is ok.

Leaving the house and its immediate environment, we now turn to our exposure further afield. This includes the car, which is part of our immediate and external environments.

Cars vary as to the EMF exposure they subject you to. Low frequency fields come from the alternator, and the cables which go from the alternator to the battery, and the starter motor and its cables. The starter motor and cables produce very high magnetic fields when you are starting the engine but these only last for a few seconds and are not a problem for most people. The alternator and cables can produce high fields, especially when you drive with full headlights at night. If you are very electrically sensitive then changing the layout of the cabling can significantly reduce the magnetic fields. See also car tyres, below.

Electronic dash panels will also produce low levels of high-frequency radiation, but these are not generally any problem - even to electrically sensitive (ES) people.

Electric vehicles can produce VERY high magnetic fields from the large battery currents and the electric motor. There are reports of significant increases in testicular and other cancers among men who regularly drive electric fork-lift trucks. The batteries in fork-lift trucks are often immediately under the driver's seat. It is important to consider the location of the batteries, cables and motor so that magnetic field exposure is minimised. Starting and stopping currents produce very high magnetic field pulses.

Car tyres are probably the largest contributor to magnetic field exposure in a vehicle. These fields are caused by permanent magnetism in the radial steel bands within the tyre and, to a lesser extent, permanent magnetism in the wheel hub itself. These fields are a by-product of the manufacturing processes. When the tyre rotates, large alternating magnetic fields can be produced. These are usually highest in the front foot wells and some people find they feel better in the back of the car. The answer is to de-magnetise (degauss) the wheels and tyres just as ships were demagnetised during the last war to avoid magnetic mines. Unfortunately large portable demagnetisers are rare.

We have been contacted by people concerned that they get **electric shocks** when getting out of their car. These are due to static electricity which is generated when people slide across seat covers as they prepare to get out of the car. Car seat covers are usually made of synthetic material, generating static electricity, which the driver or passenger then discharges by touching the metal body of the car. This can easily be prevented by holding onto the metal of the car, perhaps the roof or the door pillar, accessible through the door opening as you get out. This prevents static build-up, so there is no sudden discharge.

Personal radios used by the A.A., RAC, police, taxidrivers, etc. are usually higher powered than cellular phones. The older analogue types are likely to be less hazardous than digital ones. It is not recommended that you use hand-held sets without extending the aerial (if possible), and never use them inside a vehicle.

If you plan to use a **mobile phone** in the car, always have a hands-free kit with EXTERNAL AERIAL / ANTENNA.

Car **sensors** for **traffic** control usually use under-the-road magnetic field induction loops which are not an EMF hazard. Temporary traffic lights use microwave doppler units which point directly at the passing cars and usually in through the windscreen of the first car in the queue. Unless you make a habit of stopping in this position regularly this will not be a problem for most people as the power in the microwave beam is very low. It can, however, affect electrically sensitive people.

Police radar guns also direct a microwave beam at the car. This isn't a hazard for passing motorists but there have been reports of increased cancer incidence in the police officers who regularly hold the guns.

What else might there be in the neighbourhood that gives off EMFs? We will start with **mobile phones**, which may be as much part of your own environment as the environment around you. If you do not have one yourself, you will still be aware of the masts springing up like metal forests everywhere you go.

We don't think it is a good idea to use a digital **mobile phone** except in an emergency. There are two types of mobile phones, analogue and digital ones. There have been reports of cataracts, cancers and other effects from using the older, **analogue** phones, but most reported health effects are from **digital** phones. These effects include headaches, burning sensations around the ear, neck growths (Non-Hodgkin's Lymphoma), concentration and memory loss and fatigue. Even when just on standby, phones 'wake up' for a short time, and broadcast on full power, so the base station 'knows' where they are. The research seems to show that the smaller the head size of the user, the more likely there is to be a problem. We don't think children should use mobile phones at all, except in extreme circumstances.

However, for those people who use mobile phones, there have to be **mobile phone base station masts** for the phones to work. Nobody seems to like them as they are an eyesore. They are necessary, if we insist on the phones. Where to put them? Anywhere but here, is usually the response. The telecommunications companies want them high up, so as to achieve maximum coverage for optimum (minimum) power output.

In the countryside, mobile phone companies will look for places at the tops of hills to site their masts. In towns and cities, they will try to put them on top of the tallest possible buildings. Extra height is a distinct advantage to nearby buildings as it reduces the fields they are exposed to, as they will go over them. Failing high buildings, the companies will ask organisations they know are likely to be short of money and which will welcome the rental payment, which is usually some thousands of pounds per year. Schools and hospitals have been targeted, for this reason. No planning permission is needed for masts up to fifteen metres high. This measurement excludes the actual antennas which can add to the overall height. Only the owner of the land or property can refuse permission for the development. Tenants may not be allowed any say in the decision. School Governors can refuse permission on behalf of a school and many have done so. Unfortunately, sometimes the telecommunications companies then find the nearest alternative site to erect the mast and the school buildings and playgrounds may then be even more irradiated.

We have spent many pages pointing out the potential problems that can be created when we use electricity, or powered equipment. Now we will look at how electricity gets to us.

It is generated at power stations (which are primarily fuelled by coal, oil or nuclear energy), and then is distributed around the country to the people who want to use it. The cheapest way to transport the electricity is by means of overhead cables, supported by large transmission towers or **pylons.** The towers themselves do not give off electromagnetic fields. They have insulators to hold the wires which stops the metal tower from being electrified. It is the cables that are strung between them which emit magnetic and electric fields. The electric field is proportional to the line voltage, while the magnetic field depends on the load current. Typically, high voltage transmission lines carry high current and therefore give off both high electric and high magnetic fields.

The amount of EMFs coming from a high power transmission line depends on its particular configuration (the way the cables are strung). Power companies know which power line configurations are best for reducing EMF, but most utilities feel that the evidence so far does not support costly changes in the way electricity is delivered. Burying power lines *can* reduce EMFs, but this is not necessarily the case, as magnetic fields travel through soil, rocks and cement. Unless the underground lines are laid out in a way that reduces EMF, simply hiding the lines out of sight may create a false sense of security. Unfortunately, the best configurations for the lowest EMFs are less cost efficient for electric power companies to install.

If you live within 150 metres from the cables between pylons, you may be living in fields which could affect you. To find out how high the fields are likely to be, you need to find out what voltage the lines are and what they are supplying. Residential properties will make different demands and have different peak load times to industrial premises. Some places e.g. supermarkets, some industries, hospitals, etc., may require a 24-hour continuous supply of electricity. High power lines may need greater clearance, some low power lines may need less, depending on factors such as how large the load is and whether the load is balanced. These factors are not always easy to discover. The distances below is where the average field falls to background levels of EMFs. At these distances we strongly recommend you have the fields measured.

      120 metres from 400kV & 275kV lines
      100 metres from 132kV lines
        50 metres from 33kV lines (usually on wooden poles)
        25 metres from 11kV lines (on wooden poles)

Some lines are fine closer than this, some of the largest may need 250 metres. Some recent research done at Bristol University shows that the electric fields surrounding overhead cables cause air ionisation, attracting fine particles which can include carcinogenic (cancer-producing) particles, which are then wind-blown or carried in the rain up to 500 metres or more down wind of a 400 kV electricity transmission line.

When trying to find out what level of field you will be exposed to, the critical distance is that measured by a straight line between the building and the nearest wires, whether the pylons are on a hill above, below or at the same height as the building.

As mentioned above, sometimes **cables** are put **underground**. This reduces the visual impact, but does not necessarily remove the magnetic field hazard. The **electric** fields will be zero as they are screened by earth, concrete, sand etc.

The **magnetic** fields are very high near to the cable, higher than from overhead cables, because they are closer to you. They fall off more rapidly than the fields from overhead wires, because the cables are closer together and cancel out each other's effects more quickly. They are usually at an acceptable level by 5-30 metres, unless there are multiple cables carrying a very high load, when the distance for the fields to drop to an acceptable level is more likely to be 50 metres. If you are at all unsure, we recommend measurement of the fields to determine the field level in your particular circumstances.

The voltage carried by overground or underground cables has to be reduced in order to be able to be used in our homes, shops, factories, etc. This reduction is done at **substations** or **transformers**.

Low power substations are found about 150 metres apart in a typical urban area. So you will never be *that* far away from one. Rural areas are more variable. Magnetic fields associated with substations come mainly from the low voltage (240 / 415 volt) underground cables supplying the power to houses, factories, etc. If there is a substation very close to your home, you would need to find out where the underground cables are in relation to your property, and have the electric and magnetic fields measured, to discover if it increases the background field level experienced by you and your family. (Your Regional Electricity Company or Primary Electricity Supplier will usually offer this service free of charge if you live next to a substation). It is important to remember that fields in winter and/or cold weather can be up to three times higher than those measured in warm weather. Times of peak use, that is about 8.00 to 9.15 a.m. and about 4.30 to 6.30 p.m., will also be higher than other times of day. These times do not always coincide with the times the Electricity Company or Supplier will measure your fields. Bear that in mind in considering your exposure levels.

Fields from the substation equipment itself fall to a 'safe' level approximately 3 metres from the wall of an 11kV substation, 8 metres from a 33kV substation and further away for higher voltage substations (these are more variable, so less predictable). For the purposes of this book, 'safe' is considered to be the level at which no associated increased risk has been identified in the research done up to the date of publication.

The incoming and outgoing currents at a substation are generally unbalanced. High magnetic fields from substations have been blamed for causing cancer clusters among nearby residents.

Ideally, all currents should flow out from a source (e.g. an electricity substation) and return to the same source along two wires which run close together. The wires will then produce almost identical but opposite magnetic fields that virtually cancel out. In many built up areas the electricity companies often connect neutrals from different substations together. The reason they give is to minimise "over-voltage" conditions which might occur and damage your equipment if the local neutral becomes broken. If this does happen when neutrals are linked, everything will continue to work as usual, but the current flows back down the 'wrong' wire. This produces **"net currents"** which flow round the system and can give rise to high magnetic fields over wide areas (e.g. round 4 or 5 streets). This is a major cause of high domestic magnetic field levels and the only way to find out if it is happening in your area is to measure the magnetic fields at a peak time (say between 4.30 and 6.30 p.m. on weekdays). Fields should be _well_ below 100 nanotesla (0.1 microtesla) in the summer, and 200 nT (0.2 microtesla) in the middle of winter.

Net currents can also occur with the 'ring wiring' used in UK houses and offices used to feed the electrical socket outlets. We dislike this wiring technique and believe all wiring should be 'radial' which forces the return current to return alongside the supply current. This is covered in detail in Chapter 6.

Many substations make humming or buzzing noises when they are working. The noise level is more intrusive at night-time, when it is generally quieter. The volume of 'buzz' will be more or less dependent on the substation's loading. If a particular substation does not buzz it means that the substation is efficient in its activity, not necessarily that it is supplying less power. The sound might mean that the substation is high-loaded and/or not working properly. The magnetic fields should be measured and the cause of the noise investigated by your local Electricity Company.

Your local Environmental Health Department sets the noise level which is considered to be acceptable, especially at night. You could contact them if you believe your local substation might exceed this level.

The noise is essentially a problem of vibration. If the transformer inside the substation has loose laminations, the Company may replace it. However, a transformer costs approximately £15 - £40,000 to change, so the Company will be unlikely to do so, if it complies with the Environmental Health-determined noise levels and there are no other operational problems.

Other remedial action they could take is:-

a) to mount the transformer on rubber blocks.

b) to put a sound proofed fibre-glass enclosure around the substation.

Pole-mounted transformers can be found in more rural areas. They perform the same task as an urban substation. Three metres is usually adequate for fields from these transformers to fall to an acceptable level.

Is it safe for children to play in the garden near lines, cables or next to substations?

The difficulties arise with the words 'safe' and 'near'. The higher the voltage of the line or cable, the greater the field levels will be and the further away children should play. Electric fields can be reduced considerably by shrubs, bushes and trees. Deciduous trees (that lose their leaves in Winter) will provide less protection then, but children are likely to play outside for shorter periods of time. Magnetic fields only reduce with distance from the source. Again, bushes can be used, not to reduce fields, but so that children are unable to play in the higher fields where the bushes are growing. Be careful of trees and bushes that will make good 'dens' or 'tree houses' as that really defeats the object, and indeed will encourage children to stay put in these high fields.

We do not believe it is safe to play near high-voltage overhead lines above 11kV, especially with the new concerns about electric field aerosol effects (see **Pylons**, above, and the research from Bristol University). Evidence suggests that moving about in magnetic fields of up to 500nT is unlikely to be hazardous.

It is important not to allow babies to sleep in prams in these sort of field levels and to discourage convalescing children to be out in high fields. It is a good idea to measure garden EMFs if you have any concerns about what areas are 'safe' and what areas need to be avoided. Although research has shown there is an increased risk of illness in high fields, **most** people, including **most** children will **not** be seriously affected by them. It is important not to panic, but to take reasonable precautions.

We have been asked about the effect of EMFs on plants and vegatables growing in gardens near substations or under powerlines. As far as we know no detailed research has been done to look into this. Because it is known from laboratory experiments that EMFs affect the polarisation of water molecules, and inter- and intra-cellular communication, we would assume that it will affect any growing thing. It is unclear what the effect may be of eating a diet entirely composed of food grown in these conditions. If anyone knows of research or anecdotal evidence of such effects we will be very keen to hear.

There has been a lot of work done on the effects of geopathic stress and vegetable and plant growth. This research has been done mainly in Europe where they are way ahead of Britain in investigating these phenomena. We have found restricted growth or dying plants in areas of geopathic stress. Human health has been shown to be affected by the combination of medium-level magnetic fields and geopathic stress, especially that caused by underground water lines. It is very likely that it will affect plants and possibly the eater of fruit and vegetables so affected. We suspect that whatever effects they may have will be rather more subtle than the effects of pesticide and herbicide exposure on the eater of commercially grown produce, so it is worth keeping it in perspective. And eating organic, whenever possible.

We go further afield to consider the effects of **TV** and **Radio transmitters.** We are constantly being bathed in more and more radiofrequency and microwave signals. This will increase dramatically over the next few years with the phasing out of analogue TV signals and their replacement with digital ones. Average US city dwellers are now subject to levels 200 times higher than they were in 1980 - a figure which is probably similar in the UK. We are now surrounded by artificial radiation over one million times higher than the natural radiations at these frequencies that our relatives were exposed to in 1900. We do not know for sure if this exposure is harmful, but our reading of the evidence is that it is good to reduce exposure as much as possible.

There is not much you can do about the ambient levels around your house, but you may bear this issue in mind if moving to a new area.

Radar gives off very high pulsed fields. These can extend to several miles away in the case of long distance military radar such as at Fylingdales in Yorkshire. Microwave radar levels can also be concerningly high within about half a mile of commercial airports.

I hear a noise like a 'Hum' which I find disturbing. What is the cause?

The source of a 'hum' can be difficult to find. Hum does **not** usually come from electrical cables and equipment, although transformers do hum slightly and, if faulty, can hum loudly. Ask others if they can hear the hum, not just the people living in the same house as yourself.

A common source of hum is road noise, from major roads up to 1 mile away, resonating in bedrooms. It can usually be cured by thick curtains and other sound absorbent materials. Another source of Low Frequency Noise comes from long distance major gas pipe lines which are pressurised by large engines. This sound can travel several miles through the ground and only <u>some</u> people can sense it. It does not show up on normal noise level meters, specialised equipment is necessary.

What can I do if I am being 'zapped' by my neighbours?

Unless you have been involved in 'subversive activities,' as a result of which you have been targeted by official agencies, it is almost certain that you will not be being zapped intentionally. If you feel you are being 'zapped', it is most likely that you have developed electrical or chemical hypersensitivity.

CHAPTER FOUR
SPECIAL NEEDS

This chapter covers the equipment you may find in the homes of people who have mobility problems, hearing problems, etc.

We have found ENORMOUS magnetic fields (several microtesla) being given off all the time by some **motor-adjustable reclining beds and chairs**. Some have also had unexpectedly large electric fields. There is no excuse for these high field levels - it is just bad design by people who have never thought about possible dangers from EMFs and come from internal wiring and cheap transformers which are connected all the time the chair or bed is plugged in and turned on. It is quite easy to design such a chair or bed with almost unmeasureable EMFs other than when actually using the motors to make the mechanical adjustments. If you have one of these beds or chairs then we suggest that you measure both the electric and magnetic fields. If they are high, switch the supply off <u>at the wall</u> or unplug it when you are comfortable.

Lifts are lowered and raised on cables driven by motors. The fields will come from the motor. This can be in a separate housing at the bottom of the liftwell, or at the top; underneath an integral chair, or underneath the lift floor if the lift is used specifically for wheelchairs, and does not have an integral chair. The closer the motor is to the person in the lift, the higher the fields they will experience.

In a multi-storey complex (e.g. flats), the lift motors are much larger and if you live in the top apartment then it is wise to find out where the motors are, and either keep at least 3 metres away, or measure the fields to see how far they extend.

Stairlifts have motors mounted on the actual chair, so you are exposed to high magnetic fields when using it. This probably is not a problem as long as you only use it relatively few times each day.

A **TENS unit**, (**T**ranscutaneous **E**lectrical **N**erve **S**timulator unit), can help to exercise and relax muscles, using electrical stimulation to give rise to natural endorphins which can give pain relief. We do not consider these to be hazardous from an EMF point of view.

Wheelchairs use battery driven motors which will give off EMFs when in use, especially when started and stopped. High fields are also given off from the wires of a heavy-duty battery. If you use your wheelchair for fairly short periods of time, there are likely to be few EMF problems. If you use your wheelchair all the time it may be worth while taking extra precautions. There has been research linking extensive use of forklift trucks with testicular and other cancers. As there are relatively few female forklift truck drivers, similar research has not been done for women and the possible increased risk of cervical cancer. The longer the time you spend in an electrically moving wheelchair the more you will be exposed to high fields. It is worth getting regular medical checkups to detect any possible physical changes at an early stage.

Wheelchairs are not designed to minimise EMF exposure. To reduce your total exposure, it is possible to put a steel sheet underneath the wheelchair seat and also down behind your legs. Put an extra cushion on top of the seat.

The motors used to power **bath hoists** give off high magnetic fields when in operation, but occasional exposure (one bath per day) is unlikely to cause a problem. People operating a bath hoist on a regular basis, e.g. a care assistant in a day centre or residential home, will be exposed to high fields over a much longer period of time, and for women, there may be increased risk of breast cancer if the motor is at chest height.

As far as we know all battery-operated **personal alarms, as used in warden-controlled accommodation,** are safe.

The power used by **hearing aids** is absolutely tiny, and we do not know of any EMF problems associated with their use.

Induction Loop systems are to amplify sound for the hard of hearing in their own home watching TV, or in public places like theatres, conference rooms, etc.

Instead of using a loudspeaker, sound is amplified and transmitted using a large loop of wire wound around the room or building. This sound cannot be heard directly but it is picked up by a special loop and receiver worn by the person who is hard of hearing, and fed to a hearing aid.

This induction loop system causes quite high levels of EMFs but as they change continually with the broadcast sound, there is no evidence of any harm. In fact, one American researcher found that such varying signals can actually reduce danger from the background EMFs found in buildings, by effectively masking them to some extent - rather like music played in a restaurant making it harder to hear other people's conversations.

The next two amplified hearing systems are primarily used in people's homes rather than in public places.

Infra-red systems work by transmitting the sound signal using an infra-red beam (using a similar method to the one used by a TV remote controller), from the television to a head set worn by the person who is hard of hearing. This use of infra-red light uses very low power and is free of any electromagnetic hazard.

Microwave systems have a microwave transmitter attached to the television set or Hi-Fi system. The receiver is in the headset worn by the person listening. The headsets are safe, but the transmitter gives off high fields. You should sit a reasonable distance away from the transmitter unit. We were contacted by a special needs teacher who uses a microwave transmitter, which hangs down on the chest, broadcasting to one or more students' receivers. The units work on very low power, but as breast tissue absorbs microwaves easily, the unit would be best placed on the desk and used with the optional separate microphone. The teacher can carry the unit to different places within the classroom, but it will be kept at a distance from vulnerable body tissue.

Foot and hand warmers which are used for outdoor pursuits, e.g. motorbiking, use DC electricity to provide the heat. This will produce local field distortions, but are unlikely to have any adverse effects unless they are used for prolonged periods. Mains electricity powered units for the elderly may be a problem as they can give off both electric and magnetic fields at significant levels. It would be best to use 12 volt DC powered ones intended for motor-bike use and run them from a battery charger positioned at least 1.2 metres away from the wearer.

About 1 in 1,000 of the population are to some degree **electrically sensitive**. Electrical sensitivity (ES) can have a variety of causes. Computer monitors, and increasingly mobile phones, are believed to be the most common initiators of the problem. Symptoms of this condition are very similar to many other allergic conditions, and can be provoked by using electrical equipment or being near equipment that is being used. Providing that the intensity of the field is greater than the threshold of sensitivity (which can be very low), it will cause an allergic reaction. The threshold for sensitivity to 50 Hz fields can be as low as 25 volts per metre electric field and 30 nanotesla magnetic field. When the body is exposed to a large number of man-made ELF frequencies, the immune system becomes overloaded and starts to react with symptoms which can include flushing and blushing, palpitations, diarrhoea, muscular aches, noises in the head, pins and needles, especially in hands and feet, dizziness, fits and blackouts, disorientation, headaches, depression and persistent tiredness unrelieved by rest. Electrical sensitivity may also mimic neurological diseases such as paralysis, epilepsy and MS.

People who have developed electrical sensitivity may also experience the following:

- frequent electric shocks from objects, that do not affect other people;
- inability to wear synthetic fibres, especially nylon, due to the build up of static electricity;
- fluorescent lighting may make you feel unwell. However, full spectrum fluorescent lights are much less of a problem. We have found some early high-frequency fluorescent lights give off very high levels of low frequency radio waves (30 - 150 kHz) which can exceed 80 volts per metre at head height. These can even affect people who are not otherwise electrically sensitive;
- often feeling worse before a thunderstorm. This can be due to electric field or ionisation sensitivity.
- electrical equipment sometimes malfunctions; e.g. computers, washing machines, electric car ignitions, quartz watches, etc, don't operate normally in the presence of the sensitised individual whose body itself gives off fields strong enough to affect equipment;

We have been told that people who are electrically sensitive can find it helpful if they 'earth' themselves by walking barefoot on the grass or on concrete for half an hour a day;

There are homoeopathic remedies which can help alleviate the symptoms of ES in some people, and there are support groups which may be useful if your family or GP do not give credibility to the diagnosis of ES. Swedish Trade Unions fully recognise ES Syndrome and a number of firms now provide specially screened areas for sensitive workers.

CHAPTER FIVE
APPLIANCE LIST

Any appliance which only has a two wire mains lead (i.e. Neutral [blue] & Line [brown]) and no 'Earth' connection [green/yellow] will almost always give off high electric fields. This applies to many lamps.

Most battery / mains appliances only have two-wire connections, and also usually contain a cheap transformer which 'leaks' high levels of magnetic fields even when the appliance's own switch is off. <u>Such appliances need to be switched off at the wall, or unplugged, to remove the fields.</u>

The EMFs appliances give off vary greatly from one make and model to another. The ONLY sure way of knowing is to obtain a meter and measure them. In our opinion it is wise to minimise all exposure to electromagnetic fields.

The NRPB, other advisory bodies, and some researchers have used what is called a "time-weighted average" (TWA) to assess the amount of radiation you are exposed to because of a particular piece of equipment. They obtain this by calculating the fields given off by the piece of equipment, and the amount of time you use it and then average this over 24 hours. Although this sounds like a reasonable idea in theory, in practice, the body does not average out what it is exposed to over a certain period of time. It reacts to whatever level of exposure is **actually** there during critical periods.

The evidence does not make it clear whether long-term low-level chronic exposure is worse than short periods of high exposure. However, the evidence points towards the conclusion that you are more likely to experience adverse health effects if you are sitting or lying still in higher than normal fields for extended periods of time. The melatonin evidence, discussed elsewhere, suggests that it is unwise to have high exposure, even for short periods, in the evening. We believe that electrical appliance use in the kitchen and elsewhere should be minimised - especially if you are standing closer than a metre away from the source. Night time exposure, when you are in bed, should be minimised as the top prioriry. We believe that this is the time when EMF effects are likely to be strongest when you are asleep and your body is repairing itself.

Increasing numbers of devices are being sold which claim to 'protect' us from the harmful effects of EMFs. Most of these claims are scientifically unverifiable. Some are not measurable, but based on sound hypotheses that are concerned with the body's subtle energy fields. Some are just rip-offs. See Chapter 7 for particular devices.

Air Conditioners

Large air conditioning units are likely to be externally mounted, with pumps and motors giving off high levels of magnetic fields. They should be 1.5 metres from anything important. If you have double glazing without windows that open, your air-conditioning system may become clogged with dirt and pollutants, which then re-circulate increasing the spread of airborne micro-organisms and bacteria, making you more vulnerable to sickness. It is important to keep the system clean and well maintained.

Amateur (Ham) radio transmitters

These can emit high levels of radiofrequency and microwave radiation and should not be in the house. Most of the radiation is associated with the aerials and can extend for a considerable distance. Amateur UHF Moon-Bounce transmitters use a highly focused aerial array with extremely high power in the main beam. These arrays should be kept away from children's play areas and neighbouring houses.

Amplifiers, electric guitars and keyboards

The musical instruments are usually earthed systems and are not an EMF hazard. The amplifiers contain a transformer which gives off low levels of EMFs. Take care in its placement if used in the home.

Aquarium

The pumps that oxygenate most aquariums give off very high magnetic fields, between 3 - 400 nanotesla at half a metre. Keep chairs about a metre away from the pumps. Aquarium heaters are not normally earthed and can leak electricity into the water causing the whole tank to give off suprisingly high electric fields.

Baby alarm

Alarms plugged into the mains should be at least 1 metre away from the baby's bedhead. Battery-operated, wire connected, alarms give off virtually zero fields. The walk-about 'freedom' alarms radiate radio-frequency energy next to the child in order to communicate with the parents' listening unit and should be used with great caution.

Barbecues
These are rarely electrical and, anyway, are only used for short periods and so will not pose a problem.
Bath Hoists
The motors give off high magnetic fields when in operation, occasional exposure is unlikely to cause a problem. People operating a bath hoist on a regular basis, e.g. a care assistant in a day centre or residential home, will be exposed to high fields over a much longer period of time, and for women, there may be increased risk of breast cancer if the motor is at chest height.
Battery operated equipment
Batteries do not give off high EMFs. However, they are not energy-efficient: manufacturing them uses 50 times more energy than they will ever produce. They usually contain mercury, cadmium, lithium and other toxic, non-biodegradable metals that can affect water supplies from land-fill. Re-chargeable batteries should be used and then recycled if possible. It is better to consider your overall use of power-driven appliances, than just replace mains operated equipment with battery ones.
Beds
Metal
Beds with metal frames and bedsprings can become magnetised due to domestic wiring and electrical appliances in the bedroom, causing restlessness and insomnia. Bedframes can be de-gaussed, but places capable of doing so are scarce. If concerned, find an alternative bed-base and unsprung mattress, preferably with natural materials.
Motor-adjustable reclining
They can give off high electric and ENORMOUS magnetic fields (several µT) even when stationary. You need to weigh up the advantages of this type of bed against the potential damaging affect on an already compromised immune system. It is quite easy to design such a bed with almost unmeasureable EMFs other than when actually using the motors to make the mechanical adjustments. If you have one of these beds then we suggest that you measure both the electric and magnetic fields. If they are high, the only easy thing to do is to turn off the supply at the wall when you are comfortable.

Water beds
    These can give high magnetic fields from the water heaters and we suggest that you measure them. Waterbeds should ideally be warmed during the day, and unplugged before going to bed. A thick mattress pad or quilt will help you to stay warm on an unheated water bed.

Bedhead lights - see **Lighting**

Bedside lights - see **Lighting**

Bottle warmer
    Electric **bottle warmers** for baby bottles only give off low levels of EMFs Some only have a two-wire connection and so give off AC electric fields. Only use when necessary.

Bra
    Underwired (with metal wire) bras can act as 'antennas' re-radiating EMFs, including microwave radiation from mobile phones, into the body.

Burglar Alarm

Main control units
    These often contain 'cheap' transformers which give off quite high magnetic fields. Typical magnetic field at 50 cm. is around 160 nT, so ideally keep chairs, etc., at least 1 m away.

    They often have 'double insulated' or otherwise 'isolated' sensing circuit wires which are not referenced to 'earth' and which can therefore give off quite high levels of electric fields. If this is the case then all the wiring to the sensors and alarms will also be giving off high electric fields. If you do measure high fields coming from them you need to consult the manufacturer / supplier of the system and ask them to "reference the secondary circuits to earth". In some systems this only consists of connecting one of the wires to earth inside the alarm box, however some advanced 'tamper proof' sensing circuits will sound the alarm if this is done and then expert advice from the supplier is needed.

Burglar Alarm sensors
    Most burglar alarms use simple switch or resistive sensors on doors and windows and passive infra-red sensors for rooms and corridors. These sense the heat given off by a moving body and their sensitivity can usually be adjusted so that cats and dogs do not set them off. Light-beam sensors are rarely used nowadays. None of these sensors give off significant EMFs.

Recently active microwave sensors have been used in both domestic and commercial buildings. These usually give out low level microwaves all the time and so we do not recommend their use. If you already have them in your system then you should contact your supplier and discover how to turn off the microwave transmitters in the sensors when you are moving about in the building and the alarm is not required as they are otherwise often energised 24 hours a day, even when the alarm is apparently turned off.

Buzzes - see **Substations**
Cables
Overhead - see **pylons**
Cables
Underground

Burying power lines can reduce electric fields, but may have little effect on magnetic fields. Unless the underground lines are laid out to reduce EMFs, simply hiding the lines out of sight may create a false sense of security. Unfortunately, the best configurations for the lowest EMFs are usually more costly to install for the electricity companies.

Near the cables, the **magnetic** fields are higher than from overhead cables, because they are closer to you, but fall off more rapidly, because the cables are closer together and cancel out each other's effects more quickly. They are usually at an acceptable level by somewhere between 5 - 30 metres, up to 50 metres for multiple cables carrying a very high load. If you are at all unsure, we recommend measurement of the fields.

Camcorder

The motor generates high fields, but is well shielded, so the person doing the filming is ok.

Car

The starter motor and cables produce very high, but brief, magnetic fields when the engine starts. The alternator and cables can produce high fields, especially when you drive with full headlights at night. If you are very electrically sensitive then changing the layout of the cabling can significantly reduce the magnetic fields.

Electronic dash panels also produce low levels of high-frequency radiation, but these are not generally any problem - even to ES people.

Car Tyres are probably the largest contributor to magnetic field exposure in a vehicle. These fields are caused by permanent magnetism, a by-product of the manufacturing processes, in the radial steel bands within the tyre and also in the wheel hub itself. When the tyre rotates, large alternating magnetic fields, usually highest in the front foot wells, can be produced. Some people find they feel better in the back of the car. De-magnetising (degaussing) the wheels and tyres, remedies the problem, but large portable demagnetisers are rare.

Car Phones

Radio phones used by the A.A., RAC, police, taxidrivers, etc. are usually higher powered than cellular phones. The older analogue types are less hazardous than digital ones. Do not use hand-held sets without extending the aerial (if possible), and never use them inside a vehicle.

If you plan to use a **mobile phone** in the car, always have a hands-free kit with EXTERNAL AERIAL / ANTENNA.

Traffic sensors

Car **sensors** for **traffic** control usually use under-the-road magnetic field induction loops which are not an EMF hazard. Temporary traffic lights use low-power microwave doppler units which point directly at passing cars and usually in through the windscreen of the first car in the queue. It can affect electro-sensitive people.

Police radar guns direct a microwave beam at the car. This is not a problem for the motorist but there have been reports of increased cancer incidence in police officers who regularly hold the guns.

<u>**Carbon Monoxide detectors**</u>
- see small battery-powered <u>**smoke detectors**</u>.

<u>**Cassette player**</u>

Video cassette recorders and **players** can give off high fields if not 'earthed', which is a common situation. Portable **audio cassette players** can sometimes be put on shelves or cupboards near children's and young people's bedheads. If the player is unearthed, it should be switched off at the socket or unplugged, to ensure that the internal speaker fields do not affect the sleeping person. Often the main amplifier will have an earthing terminal on the back panel and this should be connected to mains earth. This is all that needs to be done. If the amplifier does not have an earth terminal, but instead has a three-core mains lead, then the earth will be connected internally.

Most **remote control units** use infra-red signals to transmit the control messages and these units do not produce concerning EMF levels.

CD Player see **Hi-Fi**

Central heating

Central heating **boilers** do not generally give off any EMFs apart from a short burst when the electronic ignition fires if the boiler doesn't have a pilot light (flame) which burns continuously.

Central heating pumps give off high fields close by - over 20,000 nanotesla - which typically fall to around 500 nT at 50 cm. We recommend that chairs and beds are located at least 1.2 metres away from these pumps.

If your central Heating **Timer** is electromechanical and rotates then it will give off a magnetic field at 50 cm of about 130 nT.

Hot air central heating systems have a fan which will usually be situated near the heat-source (whatever the type of fuel is). The electric motor to the fan will give off significant levels of EMFs nearby

Some **hot water radiators** and pipes that are part of central heating systems give off EMFs. This occurs when the metal pipes are carrying **'net' currents** causing high magnetic fields of several microtesla. These 'net' currents are due to wiring faults which can be either inside or outside your property and are dealt with in Chapter 6 on low EMF wiring.

Underfloor heating

Hot water pipes are usually fine but can suffer from 'net' currents as above. Electric heating cables can give off high levels of magnetic fields and can generate EMF 'hotspots'. We cannot recommend underfloor heating using electric heating cables.

Chair, motor-adjustable reclining

Some **motor-adjustable reclining chairs** give off ENORMOUS magnetic fields (several mT) all the time. They can also have unexpectedly large electric fields. It is just bad design. A chair with almost unmeasureable EMFs, other than when actually using the motors to make the mechanical adjustments, is quite easy to design. If you have one of these chairs then we suggest that you measure both the electric and magnetic fields. If they are high, switch off the supply to it at the wall or unplug it once you are comfortable.

Clock radio

Electrically powered clocks and clock-radios should be at least 1 metre from your head at night. In older analogue clocks, the motor can produce magnetic fields of up to 400 nT at 1 metre distance. Battery (only) driven clocks produce negligible fields.

Clothes Dryer

Separate **clothes dryers** which have an airer unit attached to a floor-based heater give off quite a high magnetic field, between 300 - 400 nanotesla at half a metre away.

Coffee grinder

The motor will give off high EMFs of up to 300 nT at half a metre, which drop away quite rapidly. Short periods of use should be no problem. If pregnant, it will be worth limiting time using electric appliances giving off these levels of fields at work top height.

Coffee maker

The heater will give off high EMFs which drop away quite rapidly. Short periods of use should be no problem. If pregnant, it will be worth limiting time near electric appliances giving off these levels of fields at work top height.

Computer

Most modern computers give off quite low levels of fields (up to 150 nT at 50 cm). As always, to minimise EMF exposure try to keep the computer as far away from your body as is practical.

Computer display monitors (VDU)

Extensive research has been done on VDUs and potential hazards. Old cathode ray tube (CRT) type screens can give off high EMFs and x-rays. These have been associated with a 73% increase in miscarriages and an increase in birth defects, with women who used VDUs at work. If you are concerned about VDUs we recommend the book produced by the London Hazards Centre listed in Chapter 8. The vast majority of VDU operators in the US are women and the incidence of female breast cancer has been rising steadily along with VDU use. Breast cancer now accounts for 29% of all cancers among women, and an astounding 1 out of 9 women will contract the disease. Some experts fear that long-term

VDU use will be shown to increase the likelihood of contracting cancer, and / or inhibit the ability of the computer operator to fight off cancer that might otherwise be held in check or destroyed by the body's immune system. Other less severe problems sometimes associated with VDUs are high levels of stress, headaches, anxiety, fatigue, nausea, depression, dizziness, irritability, skin redness or rashes, and eye strain.

Newer, low radiation TV type screens, complying with the Swedish **MPRII** guidelines give off far lower ELF fields (less than 25 volts/meter & 250 nT at 50 cm. from the screen). The **TCO-95** guideline levels are even lower (less than 10 V/m & 200 nT at 50cm.). It is worth checking whether your monitor complies with these standards especially if it has been given to you second-hand. This can be a problem for schools having well-meaning, but uninformed benefactors. Look for the label on the rear of the monitor. Always sit <u>at least</u> 50 cm from the front of the screen.

All VDUs give off higher fields at the back and sides. Always sit more than 1 metre from the rear of a VDU, at home, or in the office. Magnetic fields travel through walls, so watch the use of the next room. Smaller VDU's are not necessarily better, either, because the field's strength depends more on the internal design than on the screen size.

Shields placed in front of a VDU's screen do not block magnetic fields. Some of the more expensive ones (with a separate 'earthing lead') do reduce or remove electric fields, though most modern MPRII monitors do not need them. Most so-called shields just remove reflections from windows and room lights and do nothing to reduce EMFs.

Screen savers designed to blank out the screen after a short period of inactivity are useful to prevent "burn in" or damage to the VDU's phosphor coating from constant use, but even if the image is blank, the components which generate EMF emissions are still active. Similarly, dimming the display will do nothing to reduce the fields.

Some MODERN monitors are US EPA "Energy Star" compliant. These detect a shut-down signal from the computer software and do almost completely turn themselves off when not required. These take about 30 seconds to come back on line when you need them. They also need a special driver card and software in the computer itself.

When you buy a new computer monitor, switch it on in an unused well-ventilated room for about two weeks. The casing contains fire-retardant chemicals that are released in use. These can produce quite toxic side-effects in people who use them and at worst could provoke electrical sensitivity. Some companies who use a lot of VDUs and have had sensitivity / allergy problems now 'burn in' new VDUs for a couple of weeks before issuing them to employees. Also see comments above about air conditioning systems which can re-circulate toxic chemicals.

Ideally take a 15 minute break every hour when using a VDU, leaving the desk area for at least 5 minutes. It is now illegal for employers to have environments in which employees work with a computer with any visible screen display instability, flicker or wobble. (EU and UK Display Screen Equipment Regulations 1992). If your monitor behaves in this way, it is almost certainly in magnetic fields which are far too high for *you* to work in, as well as being illegal. Powerwatch offers a consultancy service to firms and Health & Safety advisers to investigate and suggest remedial action wherever possible.

Some advanced semiconductor 'TFT' colour screens are now available. These are only a few inches thick and have very clear displays. Although they do cost more that an equivalent CRT display, they give off almost zero EMFs and they take MUCH less power - thus saving office electricity and air-conditioning bills. A number of firms are now choosing these screens when purchasing new equipment.

Lap Top Computers (with LCD or TFT screens)

These give off very low EMFs. However when run from the mains adapters they can give off VERY high electric fields next to the keyboard and display (several hundred volts / metre!). Charge them up away from where you sit, and then run them off their internal re-charged batteries, or see the details in Chapter 6 about earthing such two-wire appliances.

Computer Games consoles (e.g. Playstation, SEGA, SNES, etc.)

These usually have a mains **transformer** which plugs into a power socket. They give off very high levels of magnetic fields. Unplug them when not in use. It is ***very*** important not to leave transformers plugged into the wall by children's beds as they leak quite high levels of magnetic fields all the time they are connected to the mains electricity supply. Often neither the TV nor the games controller is connected to mains 'earth' and so the hand controllers can give off electric fields of several hundred volts per metre, but it does not seem easy to predict this.

Cookers (electric ovens & hobs)

The standard electric cooker, which has an oven, grill and top plates, gives off high magnetic fields when it is operating. These can be as high as several microtesla close to. Half a metre away the fields can still be as high as 200 nanotesla (nT). Pregnant women should keep their distance, as the highest field levels can be in the area of the growing child. Prepare uncooked food in advance and keep away, as far as possible, while it is cooking.

Children's normal playing area should be at least 1.5 metres away from the front of the cooker, while the cooker, especially the oven, is on.

Research at Bristol University suggests that the average time spent cooking is about one hour a day. If you spend longer than this it is worthwhile taking especial care.

Fan assisted ovens, double ovens, toaster ovens, grills, time switches, etc. give off significant magnetic fields. Bear in mind the distance away from the body, particular areas to watch (breasts in women with family susceptibility to breast cancer; genital area for men who are concerned about testicular or prostate cancer), and whether you are pregnant. Be aware of the height and distance of time switches. The different pieces of equipment vary as to the level of magnetic field. Keep a reasonable distance away whilst they are working. Caution is needed with regard to **all** electrical appliances.

A separate hob is used on average for about three-quarters of an hour. The fields are lower than those of a cooker, about 100 nT. Pregnant women are not advised to stand in front of it for longer than necessary.

Ceramic and **halogen hobs** generate similar levels of magnetic fields as conventional open-ring electric hobs.

Hobs with **magnetic induction plates** work on a different heating principle. High EMFs are generated by the cooker on purpose, and these EMFs induce currents to flow in the pans themselves, which cause them to heat up. The top of the cooker stays relatively cool and is heated by contact with the hot pan. As high EMFs are generated on purpose, we cannot recommend this way of cooking. Some magnetic induction hobs use mains frequency fields and some use low radio frequency signals which induce currents in the pan (and people standing nearby!) more easily.

Slow cookers usually use very low power and do not pose a significant EMF hazard.

The fields from a **cooker hood** motor are high, about 260 nT half a metre away. The time spent in front of a hood is, on average, half an hour a day, so research would have us believe. Limit the time you spend in front of a cooker hood when it is dark, as high fields near head height inhibit the production of melatonin (necessary for good health - see Chapter 1), for the following night-time period.

Deep-fat fryer

The fryer will give off high EMFs as the oil is heated. Used infrequently, it shouldn't be a problem. If the work surface on which it is placed is at a height which is critical due to pregnancy or a tendency to prostate cancer in the family, take extra care. Regularly re-heated oil is more likely to cause health problems because of trace carcinogenic compounds which are generated at the high temperatures and left in the oil and which then attach themselves to the food.

Demand switches - see the end of Chapter 2, and Chapter 6

Dimmer switches - see **Lighting**

Dishwashers

Heating the water and drying the dishes is energy-intensive, generating high field levels when the machine is operating. Small children should keep at least one metre away while the dishwasher is working. The only way to be sure where the fields have fallen to a 'safe' level is to measure them. Use a timer so you use night-time off-peak electricity, keeping EMF exposure to a minimum.

Door bell

If this is battery operated then it will not give any EMF problems, apart from possible interference on AM radio when the bell is ringing. If run from mains electricity then they often have a cheaply constructed transformer which gives off high fields within about half a meter or so of it.

Electric Blankets

Underblankets and **overblankets** give off high magnetic fields that penetrate about 6 or 7 inches into the body. Some "low-magnetic field" models have been introduced, and some using DC electricity. Although these models reduce or eliminate magnetic fields, the blanket may still produce electric fields. The hot plastic coated wires release chemical fumes, which are themselves toxic.

Electric blankets commonly cause cramp. The rate of miscarriage has been found to be higher in women who use electric blankets. Pregnant women using blankets increase the risk of the child they carry developing childhood cancer. The most critical exposure time for pregnant women is the first trimester. One study [Savitz et al.,1990] reported a four-fold increase in subsequent childhood cancers in children whose mothers used electric blankets during the first three months of pregnancy, compared with an approximate doubling in risk when they used an electric blanket later on in pregnancy.

Another two studies showed up to a five-fold increase in leukaemia for children that had themselves used electric blankets.

All blankets should <u>always</u> be switched off before getting into bed. Unless you have 3-core screened cable attached to the blanket, it should be switched off at the wall. This is one place where a 'Demand Switch' is useful. Electric overblankets which are left turned on overnight are usually run from a low voltage transformer. The transformer and blanket give off even higher magnetic fields than underblankets. Do not use such a blanket if you are concerned about EMFs. A tufted lambs' wool underblanket, is a natural, safe way to keep warm.

Electric can opener

These give off high EMFs of over a microtesla (1300nT), at half a metre. Use a mechanical one whenever possible.

Electric clock

These tend to be placed quite high on the wall, likely to be more than half a metre away. Battery-powered clocks do not give off high fields.

Electric drill

Electric drills will expose you to high magnetic and electric field exposure while in use. There is nothing you can do about this and short term occasional exposure should not cause any EMF related problems.

Electric guitar see **Amplifier**

Electric kettle

Both the older style kettles and the more modern jug-type ones create high EMFs when in use. Keep the kettle at a reasonable distance when heating. Heating water using electricity can change its molecular structure. Electrically sensitive people can react badly to this change, so to neutralise this effect, stand the mug, cup or glass on a strong magnet while you pour the water into it.

Electric knife

The motor gives off fields of just over 100 nT. Reducing the number of electric gadgets you use reduces your cumulative exposure to EMFs.

Electric lawn mowers

Electric lawn mowers give off EMFs. Short term occasional exposure should not cause any EMF related problems. The motors of some lawn mowers are further away from your body when in use and so the fields your body is exposed to are lower. The evidence seems to show that occupational exposure when you are moving about is less of a risk than prolonged exposure when you are stationary.

Electric shavers

An electric razor plugged into the mains produces an extremely high AC magnetic field, as high as 20,000 - 40,000 nanotesla (20 - 40 µT) half an inch away from the cutting edge as well as electric fields of many hundreds of volts per metre. We don't know if this is worse (or better) than exposure to a 200 - 300 nT field (the level linked to increased risk of childhood cancer). If exposure to such high fields is a problem, the duration of the exposure might lessen the effects. Short-term exposure to harmful influences can produce dramatically different results to longer exposure. If this is true of EMF, (which is not as yet known), since an electric razor is used only a few minutes each day, it may be safe. The data on short-term exposure to high-strength fields is incomplete, and the use of non-electric razors will eliminate all EMF risks. The fields, close to the brain, could influence production of melatonin, if the razor is used in the evening. Use re-chargeable battery shavers. These still give off mixed frequency pulsed magnetic fields, but are likely to be safer.

Electric shower

The powerful water-heater element gives off several microtesla 30 cm away. Do not stand too close to the control unit, especially in the evening, due to the pineal gland effect.

The South West especially, (and some other areas) of England, have high radon levels. This radioactive gas, formed by the decay of uranium, can enter your water supply. It is then dispersed and inhaled in the form of hot steam from the shower or bath.

Electric toothbrush

The charger unit is unlikely to be kept, when being used, in a place which will give EMF problems. Battery-powered toothbrushes give off mixed frequency pulsed magnetic fields, the same as battery shavers.

Electric vehicles

Electric vehicles can produce VERY high magnetic fields from the large battery currents and the electric motor. Reports have shown significant increases in testicular and other cancers among men who regularly drive electric fork-lift trucks, where the batteries are often immediately under the driver's seat. It is important to consider the location of the batteries, cables and motor so that magnetic field exposure is minimised. Starting and stopping currents produced very high magnetic field pulses.

Electrical Sensitivity see Chapter 4

Electricity meter

The meter, time switches, 'consumer units' or fuse boxes, and the bulk of their associated cables give off quite high levels of electric and magnetic fields. If your meter is outside the house, the house wall will give protection from high electric fields, but not the magnetic fields. If the meter is high up on the inside wall, the fields can radiate upwards, as well as sideways and downward. It is worth remembering that walls and floors do *not* shield magnetic field levels.

If the meter cupboard is in the hallway with a room on the other side of the wall, the magnetic fields in that room will be high close to where the meter is located. Chairs which elderly or disabled people sit in for long periods of time - (longer than about an hour sitting without moving away), should be at least 1.5 metres away from the meter position on the other side of the wall.

If your meter is on the other side of a bedroom wall, as can be the case in bungalows and flats, bedheads should be sited at least 1.5 metres away from the meter position. This is especially true of anyone who is suffering from an acute or chronic immune-system deficiency. The bed of a young leukaemia victim was located immediately the other side of the wall from the meter. If the meter is high up on the wall, close to the ceiling, and there is a bedroom directly above it, it is a good idea not to place the head of a bed there.

All-electronic meters give off lower levels of magnetic fields than the older, 'spinning disc' electro-mechanical meters. If your electricity supplier wants to change your meter, you may want to ask which system they will be replacing it with, as some suppliers are experimenting with ones which give off microwaves similar to those from mobile phones. These latest design meters are intended to be remotely read without entering the house and, in some cases, to be able to adjust the charge rates for what they call 'demand-side' management purposes.

In flats or apartment or tenement blocks there is always a 'mains services riser' where electricity, gas, drains, etc., travel up the building. Areas near the riser can have significantly elevated magnetic fields which get larger towards the ground floor of the building. A doctor in the West Midlands found higher levels of clinical depression and suicide in patients who lived in lower flats next to the 'main riser'.

Electricity consumer unit or fusebox

The magnetic fields are from the layout of the cables and the currents they are supplying. Chairs and beds should be at least a metre away. There is no advantage in using circuit breakers over simple wire fuses, however it is good practice to use circuit breakers or cartridge fuses on all new or upgraded installations as they operate more reliably. See Chapter 6 for details of wiring guidance to keep EMFs low.

Mechanical **time-switches** contain a small motor. Half a metre is enough distance for these.

Energy saving bulbs - see **Lighting**

Exercise machines

These are generally not a problem. Motors (such as those used to power treadmills etc.) give off high magnetic fields close to.

Extractor fan

Motors generate high EMFs, up to 500 nT at 50 cm. If it is at head-height, reduce time spent nearer than one metre when it is on, especially when it is dark, when the fields could inhibit melatonin production.

Fan

Desk fans contain an electric motor which gives off quite high magnetic fields. Some only have a two-wire lead and are not 'earthed,' so they also give off high electric fields. For instructions how to 'earth' the fan, see Chapter 6. **Ceiling fans** contain an electric motor which will give off quite high magnetic fields resulting in a magnetic 'hotspot', extending outwards and upwards (depending on the strength of the motor) into the room above. Young children can play for long periods of time on the floor, so it is worth bearing this in mind, depending on whose bedroom may be above the fan. Check accommodation on holiday in hot countries. The room below will be fine.

Fax

They give off high magnetic fields from internal transformers. If they have only two-wire mains leads, can give off high electric fields at the keyboard.

Fire Alarm

Same as for **Burglar alarms**. See also **Smoke detectors.**

Floor polisher

Floor polishers have motors which give off high fields. Keep your feet at least half a metre away when they are in use.

Fluorescent Lights

Some of the modern high-frequency ones give off high levels of Very Low Frequency (VLF) fields (2 kHz - 200 kHz). Ordinary ones produce high magnetic fields from their ballast coils. Desk lights should be measured.

Rooms with low ceilings and fluorescent lights (as in some schools and offices) may have readings above 200 nanotesla (0.2 microtesla) at head height. In multi-storey schools with fluorescent lights, although young children may be far enough away from the ceiling fixtures, they may still be exposed to EMFs from the lights on the floor below.

Flicker and hum associated with older fluorescent lights, may be noticeable and trigger irritability, eyestrain and headaches.

'Electronic ballast' ones are better, but some of them give off radiofrequency radiation instead. Ballasts manufactured before 1978 are likely to contain PCBs, which are highly toxic and suspected carcinogens. PCBs may be released from older fluorescents, especially if the ballast is defective. Carefully replace the entire light and treat as hazardous waste.

Food processor

The motor will give off EMFs of up to 200 nT at 50 metres. The fields drop away quite rapidly and short periods of use should be no problem. If pregnant, it will be worth limiting time using electric appliances giving off these level of fields at work top height.

Foot spa

Foot spas have a motorised pump and usually an electric heater - and will generate EMFs. Feet are relatively insensitive to EMFs so there are unlikely to be any problems unless they are used frequently.

Foot & hand warmer

Foot and hand warmers which are used for outdoor pursuits, including motorbiking, use DC electricity to provide the heat. They are unlikely to have any adverse effects unless used for prolonged periods. Mains electricity powered units may give off both electric and magnetic fields at significant levels. Use 12 volt DC powered ones intended for motor-bike use and run them from a battery charger positioned at least one metre away from the wearer.

Freezer

To reduce EMF exposure and improve energy efficiency, site a chest freezer in an unheated garage. Defrost regularly for greater energy efficiency. EMFs are unlikely to be a problem.

Fridge

Keep away from the cooker to avoid the motor having to work too hard to keep the inside temperature down. A well-stocked fridge uses less power than a poorly-stocked one, since more energy is needed to cool empty space. Keep the freezer compartment of your fridge clear of ice. The motor is likely to be at the base at the back of the fridge.

Fridge / Freezer

An upright freezer is not as energy efficient as a chest freezer. The motors give off reasonably low levels of EMFs. Keep away from the cooker to avoid overworking the motor. Regularly defrost the freezer for greater energy efficiency.

Games console (Playstation, etc.) - see **Computer Games** consoles

Gardens see Chapter 3

Hair curlers / tongs

The units heating the curlers will give off significant EMF levels. When the curlers are removed for use, switch the heating unit off at the wall. If you might want to re-heat the curlers, sit away from the heating unit whilst it is still working.

Curling tongs are a self-contained, heated unit giving off quite high fields, depending on the heat setting. The metal construction will distort the magnetic field, which can increase the effects. We do not recommend their use, especially after 7.00 p.m. High magnetic fields near the head in the evening are known to interfere with the production of melatonin by the pineal gland (see Chapter 1). One study found an association between the use of curling tongs and childhood leukaemia, though this finding has not been reproduced.

Hair Dryers

These are a source of extremely high AC magnetic fields because they require high currents to produce heat. A 1600-watt model will produce 10,000 - 20,000 nanotesla (10 - 20µT) near the handle, and 1,000 - 5,000 nanotesla (1 - 5"µT) at normal drying distances (6 to 18 inches). When it is operated on its "high heat" setting, it will draw more current and generate a higher magnetic field than when it is operated on its "low heat" setting. Metal hair clips, retaining the hair in the curlers, can 'perturb' or distort the magnetic field. The fact that a hairdryer is only used for a few minutes each time, is not as significant as the fact that the user is exposed to very high fields indeed while it *is* working. Hairdressers who use a hand-held hair dryer repeatedly each workday may want to bear this in mind, especially if pregnant, being careful of the position in which they hold the hairdryer, and therefore, the position of the motor, with respect to the body. Holding the hairdryer at chest level (depending on Salon equipment design and arrangement, and the height of the hairdresser), may be problematical if the person has a family tendency to develop breast cancer. In a study carried out in 1991, the use of hair dryers was associated with increased risk of leukaemia in children.

High magnetic fields near the head in the evening are known to interfere with the production of melatonin by the pineal gland. ***We recommend that hair dryers are not used after 7.00 p.m.*** at the very latest because of this pineal gland effect. It is best to wash your hair in the morning and allow it to dry naturally.

Hood hairdryers give off a very high field; the higher the heat setting, the higher the field level. Sitting under the hood regularly may have an adverse effect. You should certainly not do so after 7.00 p.m. Any metal securing curlers, or metal parts of curler construction etc. will increase the harmful effect.

Wall mounted hairdryers which supply the hot air through a vacuum cleaner type tube are by far the best from the EMF point of view. We know these exist but are not sure how available they are in the UK.

Halogen lights

Halogen lights usually generate a lot of heat and need good ventilation if they are not to be a fire hazard.

Most halogen light fittings have their own inbuilt transformer which reduces the mains voltage to 12, 24 or 28 volts to supply the lamp filament. These transformers are usually very poorly constructed and give off quite high levels of power-frequency magnetic fields.

If set into the ceiling, with the light projecting downwards, there is not usually an EMF problem in the room being lit; but if there is a room directly above, then areas of high magnetic fields are produced in that room up to about 50 cm. from the floor. If this is a child's room they are likely to be highly exposed when playing on the floor, and possibly when lying on their bed or cot.

To avoid this, purchase low-voltage light fittings without built-in transformers and have one high quality torroidal transformer (which will produce low levels of external magnetic fields) feeding all the lights on that circuit. For instance, if you have several light fittings in a false ceiling, the a low EMF leakage torroidal transformer can be in one corner of the room, as part of the circuit between the switch and the lamps.

To minimise electric fields it is important that one side of the low voltage supply coming out of the transformer is earthed.

Halogen desk lamps usually have cheap transformers located in their base which should be positioned at least 50 cm away from your body in order to minimise EMF exposure. Although they can produce attractive 'bright pools of light,' it is important to position halogen fittings to ensure that you do not look at the bulbs directly.

Unfiltered halogen lamps usually give off high levels of light in the blue part of the spectrum and quite high levels of ultra-violet (UVA and UVB) radiation. The light from some 20 watt lamps, if looked at directly, can exceed the National Radiological Protection Board's safety guidance outlined in their "Hazard assessment of optical radiation sources used in some consumer products" (October 1991) in under one minute! For those 20 watt bulbs which have some built-in filtering, and which run at a lower temperature, it would take about 15 minutes looking at them directly to exceed the safety guidance.

One person we know developed a case of central serous retinopathy when he looked to the side of a 20 watt *unfiltered* halogen lamp for about 15 minutes, during a television interview. In this condition, the back of the retina develops a fluid-filled blister and vision is lost over this area. Luckily, he recovered his full sight over a period of 18 months; however such damage can result in permanent visual impairment.

Headphones

Headphones attached by a lead to the musical equipment are fine as long as the equipment itself is earthed. If it is unearthed the headphones will give off high electric fields.

Remote cordless headphone systems have a microwave transmitter attached to the base unit. The receiver is in the headset worn by the person listening. Headsets are safe, but the transmitter gives off high fields. Sit a reasonable distance away from the transmitting unit.

Hearing aids

The power used by hearing aids is very small, we do not know of any EMF problems associated with their use.

Induction Loops amplify sound for the hard of hearing in their own home for watching TV, or in public places, like theatres, meeting rooms, etc. Sound is amplified and transmitted using a large loop of wire wound around the room or building. This sound cannot be heard directly but is picked up by a special loop and receiver worn by the person who is hard of hearing, and fed to a hearing aid. This induction loop system causes quite high levels of EMFs but as they change continually with the broadcast sound, there is no evidence of any harm. In fact, one American researcher found that such varying signals can actually reduce danger from the background EMFs found in buildings, by effectively neutralising them to some extent.

These next two systems are primarily used in people's homes rather than in public places.

Infra-red systems work by transmitting the sound signal using an infra-red beam, from the television or hi-fi to a head set worn by the person who is hard of hearing. This use of infra-red light uses very low power and is free of any electromagnetic hazard.

Microwave systems have a microwave transmitter attached to the television set or hi-fi. The receiver is in the headset worn by the person listening. The headsets are safe, but the transmitter gives off high fields. You should sit a reasonable distance away from the transmitter unit.

Heaters

Convector heaters, Infrared heaters, Radiant 'bar' heaters and **Oil filled radiators** all give off magnetic fields close by. Be careful of chair and bed positions – half a metre away is usually adequate.

Storage - see **Storage Heaters**

Fan heaters have electric motors and heating elements with magnetic fields of about 220 nanotesla at 50 cm., and they should be kept at least 1.2 metres away from beds and chairs.

Heating Pads

Use of electric heating pads for chronic problems should be discontinued and replaced with hot water bottles.

Hi-fi, music centres, CD players etc.

These can give off high magnetic fields, but the problem is usually high electric fields. Make sure the system has a decent electrical earth connection to the mains supply. This will remove most electric fields.

Hostess trolleys

They use electric warming elements which do not use much power, so EMF hazards are minimal.

Humidifier / de-humidifiers

They work like a 'back-to-front' refrigerator. They cool the air from the room, forcing the water vapour in the air to condense out on the cooling coils and collect in a water container placed underneath. They have electric motors, with a magnetic field of 300 nanotesla at 50 cm. Chairs and beds should be at least 1.2 metres away. The water reservoir inside needs to be regularly cleaned and disinfected, as they are particularly prone to contamination by bacteria, fungi and moulds. These can produce runny noses, breathing problems and headaches.

Hums - see **Substations** and Chapter 3 for non-substation 'hum'.

Immersion Heater

The heater and its associated wiring will give off high magnetic fields. Bedheads should be at least 1 metre away from the immersion heater cupboard wall. See also **central heating pumps** which also give off high magnetic fields.

Ionisers - see Chapter 7

Iron

Electric **irons** have low fields and are not a problem. Pregnant women should try to keep the iron at least 30 cm. from their body.

Jacuzzi

Some jacuzzis have pumps and motors built in to the base which will result in your being exposed to high EMF exposure. We do not believe that short-term use in a hotel is a problem, but if the jacuzzi is in your house, then we recommend that the pumps and motors are at least half a metre away from the bath.

Keyboard - see **Amplifier**

Lift

Lift motors give off high fields. If you have a lift in your home because of a disability, the motor will be in a separate housing at the bottom of the liftwell, at the top, underneath an integral chair, or underneath the lift floor if the lift is used specifically for wheelchairs. The closer the motor is to your body the higher the fields you will experience. See also **Stairlift.**

In a multi-storey complex (e.g. flats), the lift motors are much larger and if you live in the top apartment then it is wise to find out where the motors are, and either keep at least 3 metres away, or measure the fields to see how far they extend.

Lighting

All **'energy-saving'** bulbs are fluorescent giving off VERY high localised magnetic fields. 'Electronic ballast' ones have lower magnetic fields, but some of these give off radiofrequency radiation instead!

Lights give off quite high electric fields. **Anglepoise lamps** and other metal framed lamps can give off **very** high electric fields due to the practice of wiring lights with two-core flex. Always use three core flex and connect the earth wire to the metal frame.

Bedside / bedhead lights give off high electric and magnetic fields. As two-core cabling gives off electric fields even if the light is off at the switch, screened mains cable should be used and the light should be switched off at the socket.. Re-route wires and / or use metal conduit behind the bedhead if necessary, as the cables may increase electric and magnetic field exposure to the head. If you are unsure of the levels of field behind your bed, move the bed six inches away from the wall. If you have a poor immune system or a serious illness, measure the fields and take appropriate remedial action if necessary. Lights give off high magnetic fields all the time they are switched on. Keep as far away from your head at night as is practical.

Fluorescent lights - see **Fluorescent lights**

Full-spectrum bulbs

These bulbs give out slightly higher levels of ultraviolet (UV) than standard light bulbs. Generally their use is considered beneficial.

Halogen lights - see **Halogen lights**

Spot lights

These are not normally a problem unless they are halogen lights.

Standard lamps & table lamps

Most have only a two-core mains lead feeding them - the leads give off high electric fields and should be kept well away from your body. Leads should be tied safely away, running along skirting boards wherever possible. This makes practical safety sense, for children who may spend time on the floor, and it also protects them from high electric fields from unearthed appliances, which are present even when switched off at the appliance. The wire of a table lamp should lead away on the opposite side of the base to the person sitting next to it.

Dimmer Switches

Cheap dimmer switches and wiring give off radiofrequency noise, raising the overall levels of electromagnetic pollution. Most give off quite high electromagnetic fields up to a few inches from the light switch and wires. Care needs to be taken if you have bunk beds near the switches.

Light switches and wiring

These can give off high levels of electric fields. One common cause of high magnetic fields is incorrectly wired **two-way** hall / landing **switches.** How to remedy this situation is dealt with in Chapter 6. High electric field levels towards the ceilings are usually due to modern lighting wiring practice. Wiring can be traced in the walls as it creates a line of high electric field, from the light switch upwards. When the wiring is in earthed metal conduit pipes (as originally was standard practice - and still is in public buildings) electric fields become almost non-existent.

Underfloor wiring in the upstairs floors of houses, flats, etc. gives off high magnetic fields, unless the wires are in metal conduit. This is not a problem for adults and older children usually, but for young children who can play for long periods of time on the floor, it is worth finding out where the high field levels are, then they can be avoided. Mattresses should not be placed directly on to the floor, unless you are sure where 'safe' areas are. Beds should be raised off the floor unless appropriate remedial action has neutralised the EMFs (see Chapter 6).

Loudspeaker

If the equipment the loudspeakers are attached to is earthed, they do not give off EMFs. They do contain very strong permanent magnets.

Microwave Ovens

Microwave ovens have a strong power transformer and can give off up to 30,000 nT at 15 cm. and 2,000 nT at 1 metre. They also use high levels of microwave (high frequency) radiation to cook the food. This radiation can leak out through the glass door and from around the door seals. Current regulations require that a microwave oven leak no more than 1 milliwatt per square centimetre when it leaves the factory, and 5 mW/cm^2 after a period of use. We do not know if these levels are really safe and believe microwave ovens should be used with caution. Since microwave emissions can change with normal use, ovens should be checked regularly, preferably annually, to pick up any microwave leakage from the seals. For details of a detector, see Microlarm details in Chapter 8. As microwave ovens heat food very quickly in comparison with ordinary ovens, the average time spent using one is about a quarter of an hour. Even when the microwave oven is working correctly, the microwave levels within the kitchen are likely to be significantly higher than those from any nearby cellular phone base-stations.

When in operation, ***everybody*** should stand at least 1 metre away. If the kitchen is small, children should stay out of it whilst food is cooking. **On no account** should they stand close to watch the food cooking, even if very hungry, or fascinated by some of the changes which become visible as the food cooks.

Microwave ovens have a sterilising effect, so children having major medical treatment e.g. for cancer, are often told to eat only microwave-cooked food. The medication can make them hungrier than before their treatment. It is especially important that precautions are taken for these children, and, in fact, anyone with a compromised immune system.

After cooking, food should stand for 2-3 minutes to enable the cells to re-normalise. Do <u>not</u> just warm food up. All microwave oven manufacturers recommend this. **It is important.** Heat the food or drink thoroughly, and leave to stand before consuming. This is to allow re-absorption of free radicals (which are carcinogenic), released in the heating process. A UK government report showed that 30% of microwave ovens tested did not heat mashed potato even up to the temperature designed to kill bacteria, which is another reason for taking care.

Little research has been done as to whether cooking using microwaves affects the nutritional quality of food, although there is some very concerning published information showing undesirable changes to essential amino acids and other proteins. Some people believe that there are subtle life energies in food which are affected by <u>all</u> cooking processes. Our feeling is that microwave cooking should **not** be used as the main way of cooking. This is especially true for babies, whose bodies and cellular structures are so much more vulnerable than when they are older. Baby bottles should ***<u>not</u>*** be heated to body temperature and immediately given to babies. We do not recommend a microwave oven for the cooking or heating up of **<u>any</u>** baby foods.

<u>Mixer</u> and <u>Blender</u>

The motors will give off high EMFs of up to 700 nT (mixer) and 1,000 nT (blender) at half a metre, which drop away quite rapidly. Short periods of use should be all right. If pregnant, it will be worth limiting time using electric appliances giving off this level of fields at work top height.

Mobile Phones

There have been reports of cataracts, cancers and other effects from using the older, **analogue** phones, but most reported health effects are from **digital** phones. These effects include headaches, burning sensations around the ear, neck growths (Non-Hodgkin's Lymphoma), tinnitus, concentration and memory loss and fatigue. We believe that mobile phones should only be used when absolutely essential. The research seems to show that the smaller the head size, the more likely there is to be a problem. We don't think children should use mobile phones at all, except in extreme, possibly life-threatening, circumstances.

Mobile Phone masts / base stations

Telecommunications companies like to put masts as high as possible to give maximum coverage, for optimum (minimum) power output.

In rural areas, mobile phone companies choose the tops of hills to site their masts. In towns and cities, they will put them on the tallest possible buildings. Extra height is a distinct advantage to nearby buildings as it reduces the fields they are exposed to. If high buildings are unavailable, the companies will approach places that will welcome the annual rental payment, usually some thousands of pounds. Schools, churches and hospitals have been targeted. No planning permission is needed for masts up to fifteen metres high, excluding the actual antenna height. Owners of land or property can refuse permission for the development, but not tenants. School Governors can refuse permission on behalf of a school; unfortunately the nearest alternative site may mean that the radiation is then directed at the school buildings and playgrounds, raising irradiation levels even higher.

Music Centre - see **Hi-fi**

Net currents

All currents should flow from a source (e.g. an electricity substation) and return to the same source along two wires which run close together. The wires will then produce almost identical but opposite magnetic fields that virtually cancel out. In many urban areas electricity companies often connect neutrals from different substations together. This minimises "over-voltage" conditions which may damage your equipment. If these conditions do occur, everything will continue to work as usual, but the current flows back down the 'wrong' wire, producing **"net currents"** which flow round the system giving rise to high magnetic fields over wide areas. This is a major cause of high domestic magnetic field levels and the only way to find out if it is happening in your area is to measure the magnetic fields at a peak time (4.30 to 6.30 p.m. on weekdays). The fields should be _well_ below 100 nanotesla (0.1 microtesla) in the summer, and 200 nT (0.2 microtesla) in the middle of winter.

Net currents can also occur with 'ring wiring' used in UK houses and offices to feed the electrical socket outlets. We believe all wiring should be 'radial' which forces the return current to return alongside the supply current. This is covered in detail in Chapter 6.

Nightlights

These should not be used unless absolutely necessary, because the pineal gland best produces melatonin, the body's natural anti-cancer hormone, in the dark. If necessary, have a low-wattage bulb, in a unit well away from the child's bed, keeping the wires away.

Pagers / beepers

They do not give off harmful EMFs, although there is a new generation of 'advanced' pagers which use the GSM mobile phone network and do transmit 'message received' microwave signals.

Pencil sharpeners

Electric ones have motors giving off high EMFs. They are not usually a hazard being used occasionally for short periods.

Personal alarms, as used in warden-controlled accommodation

As far as we know all battery-operated personal alarms are safe.

Personal radios and stereos

These do not pose an EMF problem when run on batteries. See **Headphones**.

Photocopiers

These can give off very high magnetic fields close to. Stand back at least 50 cm. Photocopiers emit ozone, which is affected by the surrounding electric fields. Ensure good ventilation. Toner powder is toxic when inhaled and is attracted to static electricity.

Pole-mounted power-line transformers

These can be found in more rural areas, performing the same task as an urban substation. Three metres is usually adequate for fields from these transformers to fall to an acceptable level.

Power tools

All electric power tools give off EMFs; those with motors close to your body (e.g. electric drills and hedgecutters) will expose you to high magnetic and electric fields while they are in use. Short term occasional exposure should not cause any EMF related problems. The motors of some tools are further away from your body when in use and so the fields your body is exposed to are lower. The evidence seems to show that exposure when you are moving about is less of a risk than prolonged exposure when you are stationary (i.e. in a chair or bed).

Printers

Laser printers give off ozone, which is affected by the surrounding electric fields. Ensure good ventilation. Toner powder is toxic when inhaled and is attracted to static electricity.

Inkjet and **squirtjet printers** are more economical and ecological.

Projectors

Film and **slide** projectors have motors which give off magnetic fields which fall away within half a metre. It is unlikely to be a problem, but keep your distance to avoid cumulative exposure.

Protection devices see Chapter 7

Pylons (Electricity Transmission Towers)

It is the cables, not the towers, which radiate EMFs. The electric field is proportional to the line voltage, while the magnetic field depends on the load current. Typically, high voltage transmission lines carry high current and therefore give off both high electric and high magnetic fields.

The level of EMFs coming from a high power transmission line depends on its configuration. Power companies know which power line configurations reduce EMFs, but most utilities feel that the evidence so far does not support costly changes in the way electricity is delivered.

Residential properties will make different demands and have different peak load times to industrial premises. Some places may require a 24-hour continuous supply of electricity. Factors such as how large the load is and whether the load is balanced are not always easy to discover.

Below is an indication of where the **average** field falls to background levels of EMFs. At these distances we strongly recommend you have the fields measured.

120 - 250 metres from 400kV & 275kV lines
100 metres from 132kV lines
50 metres from 33kV lines
25 metres from 11kV lines

Research done at Bristol University shows that the electric fields surrounding overhead cables cause air ionisation, attracting fine particles which can include carcinogenic (cancer-producing) particles, which are then wind-blown or carried in the rain up to 500 metres or more down wind of a 400 kV electricity transmission line.

When trying to find out what level of field you will be exposed to, the critical distance is that measured by a straight line between the building and the nearest wires, whether the pylons are on a hill above, below or at the same height as the building.

Radar

Radar gives off very high pulsed fields. These can extend to several miles away in the case of long distance military radar such as at Fylingdales in Yorkshire. Microwave radar levels can also be concerningly high within about half a mile of commercial airports.

Radio

Mains operated radios give off EMFs when connected to the mains. Keep at least a metre away when listening and unplug it or switch it off at the wall after use. Battery operated radios are fine.

Radio transmitters - see **TV / Radio transmitters**

Sandwich maker

Sandwich makers are used only briefly. Switch off at the wall immediately when finished. For many models this is the only option to being fully on, as they do not have an off switch on the machine.

Satellite dishes and receivers

They can give off high electric fields if the TV system or satellite decoder is not 'earthed' to the mains electricity safety earth. Most TVs, video recorders and satellite systems are not earthed when you buy them, as they only have two-wire mains leads. Walls will give some protection from the electric fields; windows are less effective at screening them. It is important that these systems are earthed (see Chapter 6).

Scanner

Most give off negligible fields, although some have separate mains transformers, which give off high magnetic fields.

Security Systems

Most intruder sensors should not cause EMF hazards outside your home. You should know how to switch off **microwave** sensors when you are in the garden or in other areas the sensors cover. If you do not know how, contact the installer and find out how this can be done as most systems leave the sensors active even when the system is not armed.

Sewing Machines

The motors give off high magnetic fields. Some machines with two-core mains cables give off high electric fields. Large statistically significant increases in Alzheimer's disease have been detected in machinists using industrial machines.

Smoke detector

There are many types of these. The most common type are powered by a 9 volt battery and do not give off any EMFs, however they do use a very low level radioactive source and should only be installed on ceilings and disposed of carefully if you renew them.

Smoke detectors feeding a central fire alarm system often have both temperature detectors and infra-red detectors built in. These are quite safe and do not give off EMFs.

Sockets

Electrical power **sockets** always give off electric fields. "Leakage" and / or residual damp in walls can lead to high electric field levels all over walls. For remedial treatment, see Chapter 6.

Solar heating systems

The system itself will not be an EMF hazard, except for the electric pump used to pump the water around. This could be outside or inside the house. Keep chairs, beds, etc. on the other side of the wall, at least one metre away from the pump.

Soldering irons

Those which plug directly into the mains electricity are unlikely to be a problem. Many modern soldering irons run from a low-voltage transformer / controller unit which does give off high magnetic fields. Keep it at arm's length, when possible when using it.

Spinners

The motors of a clothes spinner give off high EMFs. Bigger machines are used on the floor, draining into the sink via a hose. The field levels will be reasonably low at body height. Smaller units on draining boards, have smaller motors and lower fields, but potentially radiating more vital body areas as they are closer to the body.

Spot Lights - see Lighting

Stairlift

Stairlifts have motors mounted on the actual chair, so you are exposed to high magnetic fields when using it. This probably is not a problem as long as you only use it relatively few times each day.

Static electricity

Static electricity can give rise to electric shocks to your system, which should be avoided. Wear natural materials, and do not have carpets made of nylon or mostly synthetic materials.

Electric shocks when getting out of a car are due to static electricity which is generated when people slide across seat covers as they prepare to get out of it. Car seat covers are usually made of synthetic material, generating static electricity, which the driver or passenger then discharges by touching the metal body of the car. This can easily be prevented by holding onto the metal of the car, perhaps the roof or the door pillar, accessible through the door opening, as you slide across to get out. This prevents static build-up, so there is no sudden discharge.

Storage Heater

These give off up to 300 nT at 1 metre when charging up. Night storage heaters should always be at least 1 metre away from beds to minimise the magnetic fields in which people sleep. This especially applies to landings where fields can extend through walls.

Most (e.g. Economy 7) electric storage heaters only charge up at night (between mid-night or 1 a.m and 7 or 8 a.m. depending on whether you are on Greenwich Mean Time or British Summer Time) but some electricity tariffs allow one or two extra short charging periods during the day when the heater will also be giving off high magnetic fields. Check with your electricity supplier if you are in doubt.

Substations

Low power substations are about 150 metres apart in a typical urban area, rural areas are more variable. Magnetic fields associated with substations come mainly from the low voltage (240 / 415 volt) underground cables supplying the power to houses, etc. If there is a substation very close to you, find out where the underground cables are, and have the electric and magnetic fields measured or hire a meter from Powerwatch. Your Regional Electricity Company or Primary Electricity Supplier will sometimes offer this service free of charge to customers who live next to one of their substations. Fields in cold weather can be up to about three times higher than those measured in warm weather. Times of peak use, about 8.00 to 9.15 a.m. and about 4.30 to 6.30 p.m., will be higher than other times of day. These times do not always coincide with the times the Electricity Company or Supplier will measure your fields.

Fields from the substation equipment itself fall to a 'safe' level at approximately 3 metres from the wall of an 11 kV substation, 8 metres from a 33 kV substation and further away for higher voltage substations (these are more variable, so less predictable).

The incoming and outgoing currents at a substation are generally unbalanced. High magnetic fields from substations have been blamed for causing cancer clusters among nearby residents.

See also **Net currents**

The **humming** or **buzzing** noises that many substations make is more intrusive at night-time. The volume is more or less dependent on the substation's loading. Some substations are more efficient and do not buzz; this does not necessarily mean that they are supplying less power. The substation may be high-loaded and / or not working properly. The magnetic fields should be measured and the cause of the noise investigated by your local Electricity Company.

Your local Environmental Health Department sets acceptable noise levels, especially those at night. Contact them if you believe your local substation might exceed this level.

The noise is essentially a problem of vibration. If there is a problem with the transformer, the Company *may* replace it. However, a transformer costs approximately £15 - £40,000, so the Company will be unlikely to do so, if it complies with the Environmental Health-determined noise levels and there are no other operational problems.

Other remedial action they could take is:-

a) to mount the transformer on rubber blocks.

b) to put a sound proofed fibre-glass enclosure around the substation.

Sun beds

These give off high electric and magnetic fields as well as possibly dangerous levels of ultra-violet radiation. Many can give off five times as much UVA as would be expected from bright sunlight at the equator. They increase the risk of skin cancer, especially in fair-skinned people.

Sun lamp

These, too, give off possibly dangerous levels of ultra-violet radiation. Ultra-violet is a form of non-ionising radiation that we know causes skin cancers.

Tea maker

Keep a **tea-making machine** at least one metre from the head of your bed. It gives off high fields when in operation.

Telephone

Ordinary wired telephones are not usually a problem as one side of the telephone system is 'earthed'. However, some Electrically Sensitive people do have difficulties, as they do with most electrical equipment. In this case a 'loud-speaker phone' is usually the only practical answer.

Answerphones do not usually give off high EMFs, but most are supplied with a plug-mounted power supply transformer which does give off high magnetic fields, and should be situated at least a metre away from chairs and beds.

Car Phone - see **Cars**

Most **Cordless phones** sold in the last few years are made to the Digital European Cordless Telephone (DECT) Standard. These are more expensive than the earlier analogue phones but offer a longer operating range and most allow a number of extra handsets which can be used as intercoms or for multi-person calls.

New DECT phones are the same technology as mobile phones. We have almost as many complaints of headaches, earaches, extreme fatigue, concentration and memory loss from regular DECT users as we have from GSM / PCN digital mobile phone users. As they are charged at normal call rates, most cordless phone users spend longer on their phone calls than cellular phone users. We have only received a few adverse reports from users of the original analogue cordless telephones - mostly about brain tumours.

Unlike the analogue phones which operate at a lower frequency and do not pulse, the DECT phones emit pulses of microwave radiation very similar to cellular phones. The frequency used is around 1,900 megahertz (MHz) which is between the Orange and One2One cellular frequency band at 1,800 MHz and microwave oven radiation at 2,450 Mhz. A new frequency band at 2,400 Mhz is also being authorised.

The **base-unit** of a DECT phone emits pulses of microwaves. If you use the phone close to its main base unit then you will be exposed to two separate doses of microwave radiation. The base units also give off high levels of low frequency fields and should be located away from where you sit or sleep. The main unit ideally should be in a hall or passageway, magnetic fields **and microwaves** will travel through the wall. Any other hand-set charger units should be at least a metre from where you sit or sleep. The main DECT base unit will emit microwaves each time the phone rings but will stop if you pick up the call on an ordinary wired (land-line or cable) telephone. It emits power frequency fields while it is plugged in to the mains even when the telephone is not in use.

Cellular digital mobile phone systems are 'intelligent' and once the link is established the base station directs the handset to turn down its output to the lowest level adequate to maintain the call. In city areas and near to base stations this can be as low as 4 milliwatts peak power, half a milliwatt average. This does *not* happen with DECT cordless phones.

DECT cordless phones use fixed pulses of 250 milliwatts peak all the time. Their average power is only 11 milliwatts - but there are 100 bursts of 250 milliwatts of microwave radiation pulses next to the user's head every second. Increasing numbers of scientists believe that we are talking about electrical brain storms rather than heating effects - the regular pulsing disrupts our brain's intercellular signalling.

DECT phones also emit low frequency magnetic field pulses into the side of the user's head. These are typically up to 5,000 nanotesla in strength. Childhood leukaemia has repeatedly been associated with low frequency magnetic field levels over 250 nanotesla. We do not recommend that children use cordless phones.

Mobile Phones - see **Mobile Phones**

Televisions

Colour televisions give off up to 500 nanotesla and 100 volts per metre at 1 metre distance. Black and white televisions give off up to 200 nanotesla at 1 metre distance. In 1991, an increased rate of leukaemia was found amongst children who watched black and white television.

Television sets vary tremendously from make-to-make as to the fields radiated. Always sit at least 1 metre away from the front of the screen. The back and sides of the set also give off high fields as well as X-rays. Remember that magnetic fields travel through walls.

As well as EMFs, televisions generate static electricity. Static electricity attracts fine and superfine aerosol particles. Research from Bristol University shows that these particles can have viruses, bacteria, and carcinogens attached. They may be inhaled into the lung cavities, or may stick to the skin. Children should sit at a reasonable distance from a TV screen to avoid this affect as far as possible. The static effect persists for some time after the television has been switched off.

Ensure that you use the main switch on the set to switch off the television set. Some types of remote control leave your TV on standby and it continues to consume up to a quarter of the energy it uses when fully switched on.

These days all **TV and video remote controls** work using very low power infrared light and pose no EMF problems.

EMFs from **digital TVs** are not much different in level from older analogue models.

Digital TV receptors for both satellite and terrestrial signals can be thought of in exactly the same way as **satellite dishes** and **receivers**. There is only a subtle difference in the way the information is coded into the signal. TV reception signals are very small indeed and have no biological effect.

TV Hearing Aids - see **Hearing Aid Induction loops**

TV /Radio transmitter

Radiofrequency and microwave signals will increase over the next few years with the phasing out of analogue TV signals and their replacement with digital ones.

Stanislav Smigielski monitored the Polish military personnel for over 15 years and found that those occupationally exposed to RF and microwave radiation were 14 times more likely to develop chronic leukaemia in their old age, 9 times more likely to develop acute leukaemia and 6 times more likely to develop Non-Hodgkin's Lymphoma (NHL). NHL incidence is rising steadily in Western countries for no known reason. The estimated average exposure levels of the people in Smigielski's study were only about 5 microwatts per square centimetre, a level which can be found near powerful cellular phone base-stations and main TV and radio transmitter masts.

A major investigation was undertaken in the UK following a report by a Birmingham GP that there were high numbers of cancers close to the Sutton Coldfield transmitting mast. The cancer rates in the areas around eleven masts were looked at, and the only one with significantly more cancers than usual was the one at Sutton Coldfield. The reason for this is still unknown, but it may well have been a combination of microwave radiation and possible cancer-causing chemicals in the air. The researchers concluded that living near TV transmitting masts could *not* generally be considered an increased cancer risk.

TENS unit

A **TENS unit**, (**T**ranscutaneous **E**lectrical **N**erve **S**timulator unit), can help to exercise and relax muscles, using electrical stimulation to give rise to natural endorphins which can give pain relief. We do not consider these to be hazardous from an EMF point of view.

Toaster

Toasters are used only briefly. They give off low EMFs. Switch off at the wall immediately when finished. For many models this is the only option to being fully on, as they do not have an off switch on the machine.

Traffic sensors - see Cars

Transformers

Transformers are used whenever the mains electricity has to be stepped down to operate a piece of equipment. They are used for children's games, fish tank pumps, battery chargers, etc. They can give off very high levels of magnetic fields. Do NOT leave plugged in next to beds, especially children's beds, as it is very important not to expose children to high levels of magnetic fields while they sleep.

Trouser press / electric mangle

Trouser presses and **electric mangles** give off low EMFs and are not a problem over half a metre away.

Tumble drier

Motors give off high fields of several microtesla. Do not work close by these appliances and do not let children play in front of them, whilst they are in operation. Always keep the filter clean to improve efficiency.

Typewriters

Electric typewriters give off high magnetic fields (due to cheap transformers), and, if unearthed, the keyboards can give off high electric fields. Switch it off at the socket when it is not being used.

Underfloor heating - see Central heating.

Vacuum Cleaners

Motors produce high magnetic fields; up to 2,000 nanotesla (20 µT) at 30 cm. and up to 800 nanotesla at half a metre. The type of vacuum cleaner that runs over the floor, with an attached suction hose is better with regard to EMFs than an upright cleaner, as the motor and wires are further away from your body. Hand-held cleaners, such as those used to vacuum furniture or cars, produce high fields right next to your body.

VDU screens - see Computer display monitor

Vegetables - see Chapter 3

Video player - see cassette player - video

Washing Machines

Close to they give off high fields of several microtesla. Often pushed under work surfaces, the machines can expose vulnerable areas of the body to these high fields. We recommend you do not work close by these appliances and do not let children play in front of them, whilst they are in operation. Install a timer, so the machine can run at night on cheaper-rate electricity, when no-one is around.

Washer / dryer

A combined **washer / dryer** is similar to the two separate appliances for generating power frequency magnetic field levels. Again keep a reasonable distance from the motor while they are working.

Waste disposal unit

The **waste disposal unit** is likely to have quite a high-powered motor, which will give off high EMFs when in operation. The more organic waste that is put into the waste water system, the more expensive the water is to re-purify at sewage works.

Water beds - see **Beds**

Water filters

Jug-type water filters remove many harmful chemicals and minerals. They do not produce the subtle molecular changes that magnetic fields do. If you live in areas that are affected by the accumulated effects of years of crop spraying, with chemicals that get into the water table and then the water supply, you might use bottled water, especially for people with compromised immune systems. Many bottled waters are quite contaminated with microbes and bacteria, and can be sold quite legally, so do your research.

Some reverse osmosis filters require a pump for the membrane that separates the water molecules from other molecules. Flow rates may be slow and, along with harmful chemicals, beneficial particles including calcium and zinc salts can also be removed. It offers some protection against accidental pollution of the water supply by water authorities.

Other inline filters which store filtered water temporarily require an electric pump to release the water through the tap. These pumps give off EMFs which are unlikely to be a problem, but may affect the molecular structure of the water. Some people will be sensitive to this. It may have long-term subtle health effects on the general population.

Water heater

The heater will give off EMFs similar to an electric kettle. Height and distance from the body will vary. Minimise evening exposure time when it is dark and your pineal gland is susceptible to being deactivated.

Water softener

Some inline water softeners use magnetism to change the molecular structure of the mineral impurities in the water which create the scale that blocks pipes and causes 'scum' in the washing. Some scientists believe that these molecular structure changes can cause biological reactions and long-term health problems, if ingested. Keep drinking water separate from the water softening system, if magnets are used. All types of water filter will effectively soften water, and prevent limescale forming in kettles and steam irons.

Water supply

Electricity substations can be interconnected in a way that generates 'net' currents (for more details see Chapter 3). When electricity cables and mains water pipes share the same trenches in the street distribution system, the water supply pipe can enter a house carrying an EMF 'charge'. This causes a current to flow when the pipe is connected to the electricity earth inside the house as required by regulations. This current then flows around the house through the water pipes; central heating radiators, bathroom showers, etc., causing high levels of magnetic field. Remedial action is necessary. *See Chapter 6.*

Wheelchair

Motors and heavy-duty battery wires give off high EMFs when the wheelchair is in use, especially starting and stopping. Short periods of time are likely to give few EMF problems. If you use your wheelchair all the time it may be worth while taking extra precautions. There has been research linking extensive use of forklift trucks with testicular and prostate cancer. As there are relatively few female forklift truck drivers, similar research has not been done for women and the possible increased risk of cervical cancer. The longer the time you spend in an electrically active wheelchair the more you will be exposed to similar high fields. You could place a steel sheet underneath the wheelchair seat and also down behind your legs. Put an extra cushion on top of the seat.

Wristwatches

All watches with batteries give off significant magnetic field pulse levels every time the mechanism is activated (0.33, 0.5 or 1 second).

Zapping - see Chapter 3

CHAPTER SIX
WIRING AND REDUCING FIELDS
and finding wiring faults which cause high fields

While high electric and, especially, high magnetic fields in homes can be due to external sources such as substations and powerlines, over half of elevated fields are due to the house wiring and electrical appliances within the home. Elevated fields within the home aggravate, or may even cause, a number of chronic ill health problems. It is possible to wire buildings in ways which produce virtually zero electromagnetic fields. Often large modern commercial buildings have remarkably low (almost zero) fields from the building wiring because all the wires are run in metal trunking. We have also found enormous magnetic fields in commercial building due to currents flowing along 'earthed' pipework and metal trunking.

This chapter has been written to provide enough information for people to have their houses checked and, if necessary, have changes made to their electrical circuitry to minimise their exposure to these potentially harmful fields.

This is not intended for trained electricians. If you need further details, call our Premium Rate Helpline (0897 100 800) for more technical advice. Remember that electricity can be lethal, and all wiring installations should be checked to ensure that they are safe and that they fully comply with the UK (IEE) Wiring Regulations. It is now illegal for unqualified people to undertake electrical work in other people's properties.

This chapter refers to actual electric and magnetic field values. If you believe you may have a problem, these field values will need to be measured and you can either purchase or hire a suitable meter. Details are given in Chapter 8.

Wiring regulations are not intended to keep field levels down, although _full_ compliance with them will usually mean low field levels. Electric fields can still be high, in the order of a few hundred volts per metre in places, if metal conduit is not used. We do not recommend the use of "ring" circuits which usually feed the power sockets in UK homes as these "rings" of cable always give rise to higher magnetic fields than simple "radial" or "tree and branch" wiring which force the return current to travel back down the same piece of cable.

We believe that *ideally* power frequency magnetic fields in the home should be less than ten nanotesla (10 nT or 0.01µT) and electric fields should be less than five volts per metre (5 V/m). This is an extreme view, but in the majority of homes, levels of less than 30 nT and 10 V/m from **internal house sources** should be reasonably achievable in most of the house living areas. The electric field is the hardest to reduce due to the way many houses have been wired. The *average* total, from *all* sources (inside and outside) of mains frequency magnetic fields is around 40 to 50 nT (0.04 to 0.05µT) in UK houses.

A Report by the U.S. National Council on Radiation Protection and Measurement (NCRP) Scientific Committee 89-3 on Electric and Magnetic Fields which has members with a range of scientific and medical backgrounds called for strong action to curtail the exposure of the U.S. population to high fields. The conclusions reached by these senior scientists after several years of studying the scientific literature on low frequency EMF health effects, generally endorsed an eventual 200 nT and 10 V/m exposure limit. These conclusions were published as Chapter 7 in the book by Polk & Postow (Referenced in Chapter 8 of this book). Although opinions were not unanimous, the committee agreed to recommend a policy in which exposures would be 'As Low As Reasonably Achievable' (ALARA).

Magnetic fields

A magnetic field is produced whenever a current flows. The larger the current, the more power supplied, and the higher the magnetic field produced. In a similar way to the blood supply in our bodies, which starts and finishes at the heart, having supplied the necessary nutrients on the way, electricity uses a closed circuit which starts and ends at the local electricity substation transformer, having supplied power to consumers along the way. The supply from the substation feeds your main switch, electricity meter and fuse box (or consumer unit) where the outward and return currents should be equal.

Ideally a piece of cable has three wires in it, one of which will be a safety (protective) earth wire which should not carry any current when all is well. It is there to provide an alternative path home for the electricity if something goes dangerously wrong. The wire is either bare, with no plastic sleeving, or the sleeving is coloured green and yellow. It used to be green. A 'neutral' conductor which is connected to earth at the local electricity substation (and sometimes elsewhere, too), is used to carry the returning current. It is quite safe to touch the neutral wire (though we don't recommend you do!) as it is almost at the same electric potential as the earth, and so you should not get an electric shock from it. This wire is coloured blue in the UK. It used to be black. The third wire is the 'Live' or 'Line' conductor and this has the electric pressure (i.e. the voltage) on it and it is the source of the current used to power your appliance. **If you touch the 'Live' wire, you are likely to get a severe electric shock and could die from electrocution.** We do not recommend that you do this! This is coloured brown in the UK. It used to be red.

If the current flowing along the 'Live' wire returns back along the neutral wire in the same piece of cable, then the magnetic fields produced by the currents are equal and opposite and the magnetic fields produced virtually cancel each other out. This results in a very low magnetic field indeed, once you get a few centimetres away from the cable.

In a 'ring' circuit, the wires are laid out in a circle (more or less), starting and finishing at the fusebox. This means that current used from a electrical socket has two ways to travel to and from the fusebox (consumer unit). Currents virtually never flow equally both ways around the ring, so the magnetic fields produced do not cancel, and the wires then radiate these higher magnetic fields through the wall into the adjoining room(s).

An earthed metal conduit (wires in metal pipes) system, with radial wiring and no wiring and equipment faults, will always produce the lowest fields. If Earth Leakage Circuit Breakers (**ELCB**s) are used on the main safety protective earth wire at the fusebox / consumer unit and Residual Current Circuit Breakers (**RCB**s or **RCCB**s) are used instead of fuses, any significant imbalance in Line & Neutral currents (i.e. any **Net** currents, which will almost always raise magnetic field levels) will cause the circuit to trip out and indicate a fault.

If **radial wiring** is used instead of the usual ring circuits for power, then the magnetic fields from wiring within the house should add virtually nothing to the ambient levels from external sources, and for this reason this is the best method to use. Radial wiring is where all wiring circuits start at the consumer (fuse) box and only provide one path for the current to flow to the sockets and back again, using the same cable. Radial wiring *even without metal conduit* will produce virtually no magnetic fields.

Magnetic fields are associated with *all* electrical appliances, some giving off levels considerably higher than those found under even the most powerful overhead transmission lines. Luckily, fields from transformers and motors in such devices fall off quickly with distance, and a distance of about a metre or so is usually sufficient to bring the magnetic field down to a 'safe' level. This is because magnetic fields from transformers and motors usually fall off with the 'cube' of the distance; i.e. if you are twice the distance away, you will only experience one-eighth of the field; if you are three times the distance away, you will only experience one twenty-seventh of the original magnetic field level.

Magnetic fields from balanced current flow in wires fall off more slowly, at about the square of the distance; if you are twice the distance away from the wires, you will experience one-quarter of the field; if you are three times the distance away, you will experience one-ninth of the original magnetic field level.

Magnetic fields from unbalanced currents fall off slower still, linearly with the distance; if you are twice the distance away then you will experience half the field, if you are three times the distance away then you will experience one third of the original magnetic field level.

This is why you should always try to ensure currents are balanced within any one cable.

Background magnetic fields should still generally be below 40 nT (0.04µT) further than about a metre from most active appliances. Even an 8 kW (35 amp nominal) electric shower should only produce about 50 nT at one metre distance.

Electric Fields

These are produced by a wire having a voltage on it with respect to earth, and here a metal conduit system effectively provides an electrical screen around all such wires. However, the electric field from a three core (twin & earth) cable falls off fairly rapidly and, by careful routing, fields in critical areas (such as beds) can be minimised even with normal unscreened cable. They will always be higher than when screened (or metal conduited) wiring is used because, if not screened, some of the voltage always leaks into the building structure. Ideally you should use earthed metal conduit piping to carry the cables as this will eliminate the electric fields from the cable. Mineral insulated cables (e.g. Pyrotenax) are screened by their metal outer covering, but are very expensive to use and require extra skill.

There is suitable, reasonably priced, screened flexible cable now available, intended for eliminating electrical interference in industrial and commercial use, which can be used instead of conduited cables provided the screens are carefully and effectively terminated. This is most suitable for rewiring an existing non-conduited house.

If radial circuits are used and fitted with **demand switches** then this eliminates electric fields from circuits which are not actually supplying power.

A common cause of elevated electric fields is from the wiring of lighting circuits. It is not always obvious that these are the source, and care needs to be taken interpreting electric field readings taken with hand-held meters. To track down the source it is worth referencing the meter to a known good electrical earth - it can then easily be used to pinpoint the live sources. Otherwise it is easy to become confused as electric fields can travel up your legs from the floor and then return to a nearby earth - such as a radiator. You can then apparently get a high electric field FROM the radiator, when it is actually coming up though your body and using the radiator to return back to its source.

What are normal domestic levels?:

When you have completely switched off your home supply at the main fuse box:-

Ideally, magnetic fields should be less than **10 nT** ($0.01\mu T$) and electric fields should be less than **2 V/m** when you are more than 2 metres from the electricity meter. This is not achievable in most houses not wired using metal conduit.

Take measurements at the four corners of your home, on all floors. These readings represent the ambient background due to external wiring and currents. In towns and apartment blocks, the ambient electric field should still be comfortably below 10 V/m, but there is likely to be a higher background magnetic reading. If this exceeds 40 nT, then the cause should be investigated as it should be possible for your local Electricity Company to reduce this level, if they are willing to do so. Their underground electricity supply cables should not produce high magnetic fields in your house, but they often do, due to the way the companies interconnect them. This can be corrected, but companies are often reluctant to do so, as they don't cause *them* any problems.

Switch on all the household circuits. The fields will usually rise.

Electric fields in most areas should still be under 10 V/m. They will rise towards any wiring, and often towards the ceiling, when even in new houses it can be 50 - 100 volts / metre at head height, especially near light fittings.

These fields can almost always be reduced, and if a determined effort is made, brought down to less than **30 nT** and **10 V/m** over most of the living areas. In one fairly new 'government' erected building in Cambridge which is full of high-tech electrical equipment, I have measured the fields as being generally less than **40 nT** and **5 V/m**. This building uses good wiring practice and metal ducting and conduits.

Lighting Circuits

These are often a significant cause of elevated **magnetic fields**, either due to sharing Line feed wires or Neutral return wires, and thereby causing loops, or VERY COMMONLY by un-trained DIYers wiring circuits on stairs and landings. Here we have found double switching arrangements which have been installed without using the correct three core plus earth cable which is required to enable all the currents to come through the same lighting circuit. Instead, the lamp is fed with an un-switched upstairs Line, and returned to a downstairs lighting circuit Neutral (or vice-versa). In both cases, (which are illegal if the circuits are separately fused, but not all that uncommon), large loops are formed causing unusually high magnetic fields when the lights are switched on.

Fields from lighting circuits are often aggravated because the Line has been taken to the ceiling roses without the Neutral and/or earth, and the Neutral has been sent to the switches. This is not correct, and results in long runs of wiring sitting at 240 volts a.c. with respect to earth. The

Line should always be switched, and all new lighting circuits nowadays have to use twin & earth cable, so there is always a wire at earth potential in each cable run which helps to reduce the electric fields slightly.

However the very distributed nature of the lighting circuit wiring around the house does mean that *most* electric fields come from this source. The electric fields can be virtually eliminated by running the wires within earthed metal conduit, or using screened cable.

Ring Main Circuits

Although this is the way to wire power circuits preferred by electricians in the UK, it often causes elevated magnetic fields even when the wiring passes the UK (IEE) Wiring Regulations tests. Ring circuits were originally introduced to save on wire size and to avoid load dimming when high loads were taken from the far end of a simple radial circuit. The Ring circuit takes both ends of the three-core wire back to the same fuse so that current can flow either way around the circuit. This enables wire, which would otherwise have to be fused at 20 amps to be uprated and fused at 30 amps. However, nowadays relatively few electrical loads are that high and we believe that the EMF disadvantages of the Ring circuit outweigh any other possible advantages.

In practice once a ring circuit is installed, many people do not bother to check the loop resistances when just replacing, say, a single socket with a double socket. It is not-very-competent DIY work which usually causes most problems!

If ring circuits have to be used (and most houses will already have these) then, to achieve low E.M. fields, it is vital to have all the wiring connections as low resistance as possible, and <u>for the loop resistances to be accurately checked each time any maintenance work is carried out</u>.

In many cases it is possible to split the ring into two radial circuits (serving 2 or 3 different rooms each) and protect both circuits at 20 A without any actual new wiring other than an extra "fuse" position. **This arrangement will always give lower magnetic fields than an equivalent Ring system.** The maximum number of sockets for a given floor area and cable size and length are set out in the IEE Wiring Regulations, but in most houses that we have seen it would be legal to split the circuit in this way.

Once a ring circuit has been split this way Residual Current Circuit Breakers can be used instead of fuses to continuously monitor the current balance in the Line and Neutral pairs and so prevent fault conditions occurring which would produce elevated magnetic fields.

Magnetic fields due to system faults

The main cause of these is due to mis-wiring connections, or from neutral / earth shorts which cause Net currents and hence raise field levels. If an Earth Leakage Circuit Breaker (**ELCB**) is used on the main safety protective earth at the main electrical panel (usually by the electricity meter or consumer fuse box) this will guard against significant stray earth currents (they usually trip at 0.03 amps).

Elevated magnetic fields are also caused by stray earth currents due to faults in other buildings (or apartments in blocks of flats). These can travel back for quite long distances to the nearest Neutral / Earth connection (bonding) point, often through metal water and / or gas pipes. This can give rise to generally elevated ambient magnetic fields which change slowly with distance. These fields can easily be several microtesla (i.e. hundreds of times higher than usual).

Magnetic fields from these 'net error current' sources fall off slowly with distance. Within the loop the change with distance can be very small, but generally levels will be inversely proportional to the distance from the source. Take a reading half a metre from a suspected source. The field at one metre from a net source will be about half the value measured at half a metre. If the loop is very large due to an external fault, then the magnetic field changes very slowly with distance.

If the error current is entering your house on a water or gas pipe and leaving it on the electrical earth, then you will need to have a short length of plastic water or gas pipe inserted where the pipe enters the house. This is quite a common problem where the pipes and electricity supplies come into the house in different places. Remember, it is a legal requirement that all pipes within your house are electrically bonded to the protective safety electrical earth wire.

Screened mains cable

We recommend Type CY flexible power control cable - copper braid screened (made by RAYDEX and some other firms). This is available from RS Components and Farnell among other distributors, and your local electrical shop should be able to order you some.

This is rated for full UK mains voltage and is available in various sizes and ratings, coloured grey. Unfortunately, we have not found a suitable non-pvc screened cable.

It is not easy to use screened cables safely without experience, special tools and heat-shrink sleeving. Special metal screen-clamping glands are available for use when connecting to metal mounting boxes for sockets and switches, as an alternative to using the heat-shrink sleeving (HSS) if preferred. <u>The screen should be connected to earth at one end of each piece of cable only.</u>

Wires *may* be "screened" by wrapping them in *earthed* conductive foil, but a far better solution would be to **have earthed metal conduits installed, or use the correct screened cable which is capable of carrying the mains electricity voltage.** <u>Screened "audio cable" is NOT suitable and not safe to use!!!!</u>

Demand switches

These can be fitted in consumer boxes and wired in series with the circuit breaker or fuse. They use a low voltage to sense if a load is switched on - if it is, they switch on the mains. They shouldn't really be needed if metal conduited or screened cables are used in your installation, but can be useful for remedial electric field reduction.

Will copper or lead sheeting reduce electromagnetic fields?

Power-frequency **magnetic** fields will **not** be reduced by copper or lead sheeting. If the sheets are earthed, they will reduce **electric** fields.

Magnetic fields can only be effectively shielded using high permeability steel sheeting. It is very difficult and expensive to shield large areas such as living or working spaces. It is almost always better to prevent the fields from being generated in the first place.

Aluminium Foil

Electric fields can be greatly reduced by pasting strips of *earthed* aluminium cooking foil onto walls and ceilings, and laying underneath bedroom carpets, near wiring runs. See appendix 2. You can decorate over, or lay carpet over, these earthed foils.

Mumetal

Mumetal is an alloy of nickel, iron, and various other trace metals which is magnetically permeable, meaning that it is a good conductor of magnetic lines of force. The percentage of each element in the mumetal affects its performance, as does the thickness and method of manufacture. While mumetal can reduce magnetic fields if installed properly, it cannot block all the radiation in the same way that lead blocks out X-rays.

The Earthing of electrical appliances with two-wire mains leads

Many electrical appliances now come with two-wire mains leads or adapters and are often described as being double-insulated. This is done for a variety of reasons, including protecting against electric shock. It is cheaper to cover metal objects in plastic than it is to ensure good electrical earthing of exposed metal parts. Also, if you are holding a plastic object it doesn't provide an electrical return path to earth in the most unlikely event of your also happening to touch a 240v live electrical conductor, so you will not get a severe electrical shock.

The downside is that the 'workings' of all these appliances tend to 'float' to half the electrical supply voltage (i.e. to about 120 volts ac) and this causes them to radiate very high electric fields (often several hundreds of volts per metre nearby).

The worst offenders that we have found are televisions, videos, electronic organs, electric typewriters, some Hi-Fi units, portable computers when run off their mains adapter / charger units, and battery chargers.

Most of these can be cured of giving off high electric fields by taking an 'earthing' wire from their mains plug to an exposed screw or piece of metal on the appliance.

In the case of an organ, or Hi-Fi unit, the braid screen of one of the audio cables is normally suitable as this is connected to the '0 volt' rail inside the unit.

In the case of a television, the braid (or outside of the co-ax connector) of the aerial lead usually makes a suitable connection point.

As the television and video recorder are usually connected together it is not necessary to earth both units.

In the case of the portable computer, any metal connector shell on the back of the computer will do. It is often convenient to use a 'crocodile' clip on the earth lead so that it is easy to attach and detach when you need to move the computer. It is also possible for a qualified electronics engineer to modify the mains charger unit so that it has a three-wire mains lead and the internal 'zero volt' power supply line is connected to the electrical mains safety earth.

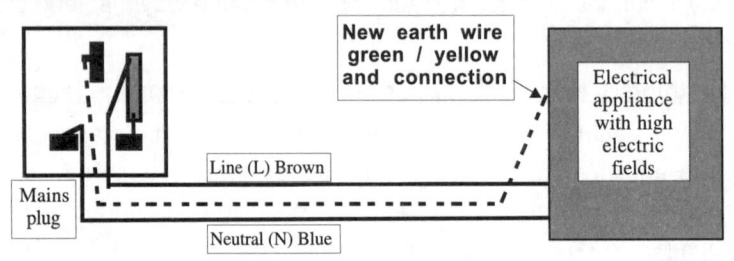

[Diagram: Mains plug connected via Line (L) Brown and Neutral (N) Blue to an Electrical appliance with high electric fields. A New earth wire green / yellow and connection is shown between them.]

Fields from transformers and motors etc., fall off approximately with the cube of the distance, i.e. the field at twice the distance should be about one eighth of the value. There is little you can do to reduce these other than use low-field designs (e.g. torroidal transformers) or increase the distance between you and the source. Steel magnetic screening can be used at the equipment but is rarely economic to do this other that at the time of the manufacture of the appliance.

CHAPTER SEVEN
PROTECTION DEVICES

Increasing numbers of devices are being marketed which claim to 'protect' us from the harmful effects of EMFs. Most of these effects are scientifically unverifiable. Some are not measurable, but are based on sound hypotheses that are concerned with the body's subtle energy fields. Some are just rip-offs.

This is not meant to be an exhaustive list. As it is impossible to judge the effectiveness of some of the subtle effects on the body's bioelectromagnetic systems, we advocate the guideline of the 60-day rule. If a company believes in its products, it should be prepared to offer a 60-day trial at least, and your money returned, less a small handling charge, if you are not satisfied. Try the product; if it works for you, keep it; if it doesn't, return it.

Often your own body is the only reliable judge as to the effectiveness of a particular device.

A - Nox EMF Bioshield

This consists of two plastic 'mini-bulbs' filled with concentrated solutions of rare-earth salts which *"react in a counter-phase mode as passive resonators to eliminate the harmful effects of TV and computer monitor EMF emissions"*. The bulbs are fixed to diagonally opposite corners of the monitor. They are claimed to remain effective for 8 hours use each day for a minimum of 2 years. There have been a number of scientific papers produced showing that they have a helpful effect on people's health. Available from Feng Shui International 07000 336 474.

Anti-Rad - see **Mobile phone shields**

Bioshield Pendants

Over 20,000 of these have apparently been manufactured and sold by the US-based Bio-electrical Shield Company over the last 8 years. Its inventor, Charles Brown, a chiropractor, developed the shield after *"voices in his head"* told him how to configure the crystals in a *"magical array which will ward off harmful rays from computers, mobile phones and electrical equipment"*. It is also said to protect against the harmful energy of other people. They vary in price from about £100 to £550. We can find no scientific basis for the claims made, nor any properly conducted trials.

They received considerable UK publicity after Cherie Blair was pictured wearing one.

Cactuses

It is said that **Cactuses** help in a room where computers are used. The spines on cactuses can attract charged ions, and therefore can change the ionisation levels in the room; however, the cactuses themselves need to be discharged. This is a problem, and they will become ineffective after a while. Theoretically, a wire taken from inside their pot to a local mains electricity earth or a bare metal water pipe would allow the charge they collect to leak safely away. But you need to ask yourself: *"am I being fair to this cactus?".*

Crystals

It has been suggested that crystals have the capacity to change many types of energies. Quartz crystals are used for all sorts of scientific purposes, mainly for their electrical resonance properties. Certainly crystal resonances can affect the electromagnetic energies nearby them ~ however this is as likely to be unhelpful as it is to be beneficial.

Diamonds (a special form of crystal) are believed to affect the energies of the owner or wearer due to the silicon impurities within the diamond. It is clear that they do have some effects. What is unclear is at what level these effects take place, and whether they are beneficial or not. Some diamonds seem to bring 'bad luck' to a succession of owners. It is worth bearing in mind that as the popularity of crystals increase, there are unscrupulous crystal miners who are devastating natural areas to obtain them to satisfy the market demand. If indeed crystals have a beneficial effect on the geology of which they are a part, we may be doing untold harm in removing them. There are better ways of protecting yourself from stress, whether it be man-made or geopathic.

Cybercap

This is a baseball-type cap made of high quality radiofrequency screening material and is available with an attachable rear piece which covers the back of the wearer's neck. Screening really only works if you completely surround whatever you are trying to screen. It then acts like a Faraday Cage and no radio-frequencies will be able to get in. However, if you just partially cover the thing you are trying to screen, then the material can resonate with the incoming energy and actually increase your exposure levels. It is a good conversation opener, even if it doesn't screen the wearer from RF very well. Some wearers have reported that they help to prevent headaches when using a computer.

EM Power Disc

This is distributed by a small UK-based organisation near Manchester. It doesn't seem to have any real electromagnetic field associations.

Empulse

Originally called **Medigen.** It is worn as a pendant and contains a small microprocessor which is programmed to produce small low frequency magnetic field pulses. It is provided by a practitioner who will measure your brainwave energies and determine if you have some frequencies missing, or only slightly present. The pendant will then be programmed with these and you wear it for a month or two before being re-examined.

It was originally developed to treat migraine, and has since been found to help a wide variety of other conditions, including ME in some sufferers. Like most treatments, whether traditional from the NHS, private mainstream medical practitioners, or complementary practitioners, its effectiveness varies considerably from patient to patient.

The Empulse is part of a process of treatment, and cannot be bought 'over the counter' as it needs to be individually programmed after your brain wave frequencies have been measured. For consultations:-

Dr David Dowson. Phone No. Bath   01225 874 075 (a.m.)
                             Reading   0118 945 2303
MDI Ltd, 17 Owen Road, Diss, Norfolk. 01379 644 234

Ionisers

Some negative **ionisers** contain a cheap transformer and give off high magnetic fields. It is a good idea to measure the field levels given off, before purchase. It is not clear which ones produce lower fields. Some only have two-wire mains leads and also give off quite high levels of electric fields. It is worth making sure that they are at least one metre away from a usual sitting or sleeping place, especially if you are uncertain of the field levels.

Air contains both negative and positive ions. Outside in the country there is a natural electric field between the earth and the ionosphere which causes an excess of negatively charged oxygen ions near to the ground (typically 300 - 1000 negative ions per cubic centimetre). Inside buildings this decreases and sometime even an excess of positive ions builds up. This often triggers restlessness, anxiety, depression, eye troubles, headaches and nausea.

Whilst many people find ionised atmospheres more pleasant to work in, this is not true of everyone. Some people find it makes them feel very uncomfortable. It is worth trying one out before you invest in one. Beware of devices just called "ionisers" - we have an example which generates both positive and negative ions in equal quantities and also has an option to generate (toxic) ozone. This does not do the same job as a modern 'negative ioniser'.

MagneTech

Produced by Dulwich Health, some people love them and others hate them. We believe the Magnetech uses permanent magnets rotated by a motor. This is really a magneto-therapy product rather than something to help protect you from EMFs. See also **RadiTech**.

Max Stress Controller

The **Max** Stress Controller is a small, battery operated, device about the size of a cigarette lighter. It operates by putting out low level magnetic field pulses from 1.6 Hz (pulses per second) on the slowest setting to just under 30 Hz on the fastest. It costs about £80 in the UK and has had some celebrity backing. There is some solid scientific work which shows that such low frequency signals can affect brain function. It is quite possible that this could be used to reduce stress or help with sleep problems as their literature claims.

Mecos

This is a small (about 60 x 60 x 10 mm) extremely low frequency magnetic pulse generator which is powered by a 3-volt battery. It generates 6 frequencies between 3 and 21 Hz (cycles per second) and was the result of many years of development of Schumann Wave devices by Dr Wolfgang Ludwig, a biophysicist from Tübingen, Germany. This does have a basis in scientific research, but it is not clear if it is still available.

Medicur

This is another development of Dr Ludwig's (see **Mecos** above). It is a small rectangular box, powered by a small 9-volt battery, which can be set to give out low frequency magnetic pulses at 3, 7.8 or 20 Hz (pulses per second). We are told that they are in widespread use throughout Europe, and a number of UK NHS and private hospitals have been using units.

The units are available for about £200 from Pure Initiative in Derbyshire (01332 882 402) with a 90-day money back guarantee. They claim that it can help with a wide variety of adverse health conditions (i.e. general pain reduction, inflammation of eyes, nose, and throat; stiffness of muscles, sore tendons, haemorrhoids, arteriosclerosis, phlebitis, Reynaud's Disease, psoriasis, acne, insect bites and stings, allergies, Chronic Fatigue Syndrome, cystitis, painful periods, eczema). The list seems very diverse and extensive.

Try it, and see if it works for you. Their money back guarantee is genuine and honoured if the Medicur does not help.

Medigen

This was originally developed by electronics engineer and migraine sufferer, Steve Walpole. It is worn as a pendant and contains a small microprocessor which is programmed for individual wearers to produce small low frequency magnetic field pulses.

The firm has been subject to some forceful take-overs but the Pendants are still available. The name has been changed to **Empulse** and more details are given above under that name.

Microshield - see Mobile phone shields

Mobile phone shields

BBC1 TV Healthcheck watchdog tested a hands-free kit, a Microshield case and a AntiRad75 case, both at an Electromagnetic Compatibility test laboratory and then in a different way at the National Physical Laboratory (NPL) using a phantom head filled with 900 MHz 'liquid brain' and a sophisticated electric-field probe inside the 'liquid brain'. Internal brain tissue does not have any nerves or ability to feel pain. Only the external head skin and tissue and the meninges just under the skull which hold the brain in place can have any sensation of feeling.

The NPL tests basically measured an analogue of SAR (Specific Absorption Rate) - i.e. the internal heating effect. The UK National Radiological Protection Board state that they do not believe that this small amount of heating is likely to cause any health problems as the level is well below their safety limits. For the hands-free kit tests the phone was placed in a jacket pocket and so chest and heart areas would be getting the internal radiation instead of the head.

The Microshield case lowers the SAR (i.e. the heating rate) into the inside of the head but is poor at reducing the electric field hitting the ear and the side of the head. Memory effects are likely to be due to microwave SAR energy beamed into the head, or the low frequency magnetic field pulses from the battery current surges in GSM digital phone handsets, which are not significantly reduced by any cases that we are aware of.

The AntiRad case stopped about 85% of the external electric field hitting the head and ear but was poor at reducing the internal heating energy. Headaches, ear-ache, skin-burning sensations, eye-tics and dizziness are more likely to be due to external microwave electric fields.

We have talked with a number of users of both makes of shielding cases who claim they stopped, or at least greatly reduced their adverse reactions. So, like all EMF issues, it is obviously very complex and still needs further research.

We believe that there is no completely safe way of holding a microwave transmitter to your head and, even when using a screening case to reduce the radiation, call times should be kept as short as possible.

Microshield   (0181 363 3333)

This is probably the most tested of the shielding cases. The UK NRPB repeats the Phone Industry line that the case makes the phone increase its output power and so makes matters worse, or at least no better. It is clear that they have not tested one in practice.

The 'Microshield' case works by sliding a spring metal strip up the side of the antenna and this does make the phone increase its power. A standard GSM handset can control its peak output power in 12 steps from 2 Watts down to 0.008 W.

The Microshield case has been tested by many independent laboratories including ones in the UK, Russia and Australia and has been found to significantly reduce the Specific Absorption Rate (SAR) level in a phantom human head. The latest two laboratories in the UK that have tested it are BT Mobile (an industry lab) and the National Physical Laboratory (in two separate sets of tests paid for by the BBC and by the Sunday Mirror). NPL found that the Microshield case reduced the radiation by up to 90 % when the phone was already operating at full power, and in the 'worst case' when the phone increased its power from operating at a low level, it still reduced the final SAR in the meningeal layer of the phantom head by about 25%.

Anti-Rad   (01458 441021)

At the EMC laboratory, the AntiRad75 stopped about 85% of the external electric fields which are likely to be a major cause of the most common complaints of headache, ear-ache, skin-burning sensations, eye-tics and dizziness. They have also confirmed these results with some further tests by Exeter University staff.

Protector

This is similar in conception to Anti-Rad but includes a large flap of material which folds up to cover the side of the user's head and which shields it from the microwave electric field from the antenna. This product has been tested by reputable independent laboratories and does work.

Ray-a-Way

A small ferrite button to attach to the phone. Cheap, but a waste of time as regards radiation reduction.

Tecno AO

See also the main entry for **Tecno AO**. While the firm itself and Montpellier University have produced some strong evidence in terms of scientific results in protecting chick embryos, we remain sceptical that attaching a small device, which does not even try to screen the radiation, to the side of a cellular phone handset would be helpful. The makers claim that the VERY low levels of ELF signals that the device is stimulated into emitting, strengthens living biosystems against any harmful effects of electromagnetic radiation. I would be tempted to use this in addition to one of the screening cases that are known to work.

Wave-Buster

A small ferrite button to attach to the phone. Cheap, but a waste of time as regards radiation reduction.

Neutralising undersheet

This goes on the bed, under the mattress. It is fitted with an earth wire connected to a socket. *Any* earthed conductive material layer will serve for this purpose, as will carefully earthing a metal bed frame. This would be useful in conjunction with other measures to reduce the electric field in a room to avoid charge build up on a person lying on the bed. If used in a room with 'normal' a.c. mains electric fields, all it will do is attract more fields to the person! Use this device with careful thought.

Plants

NASA researched ways of cleansing the air in space capsules. They found that several ordinary houseplants have the ability to cleanse many of the most common pollutants from the air, including formaldehyde. They do nothing to protect you from most EMFs, although they can help to reduce electric fields. They are:-

Peace lilies (*Spathiphyllum Wallisii*). This is very easily grown. Even we can grow them! Also spider plants (*Chlorophytum Elatum*), which are very productive indeed. There are other less well-known plants that also have this effect. As well as filtering the air, plants increase the oxygen content, improve humidity and negative ionisation.

Protector - see **Mobile phone shields**

Quantum-Magnetica

The literature contains vague pseudo-scientific waffle. They claim the energies their range of electronic boxes emit will correct the fundamental problem of random, chaotic flow of electrons within an electrical current. They make the electron flow become more coherent and orderly by applying ERT, or Electromagnetic Resonance Technology. "The result is an electromagnetic field that radiates orderliness and coherence into the environment". The boxes can "clear" quite large areas.

They cost from about £400 upwards. It is not clear if they offer a money back guarantee period. 01695 731 473.

Q-link

The Q-link pendant is manufactured by Clarus in the USA and distributed quite widely. They produce lots of scientific gobble-de-gook that can look impressive to the general public. We bought and tested one and then destructively took it apart.

They claim it is a microchip and a resonant circuit. In fact it is a coil, connected to nothing and a small single-sided printed circuit board with a pretty gold plated pattern on it and what looks like a surface mount capacitor mounted on it. When we removed it, it turned out to be a surface mount shorting link soldered to two copper pads which were not connected to anything else. The unit had no resonances between 1 Hz and 1000 MHz. Absolutely of no possible EMF protection value as far as we can understand, although the firm which sells them tell us that they have many satisfied customers and offer 90-day money-back terms.

Raditech

Designed and sold by Dulwich Health to counteract 'geopathic stress'. Early models gave off high levels of mains frequency electric fields. Recent models seem to have overcome this problem. They definitely affect the subtle energies within a house which can easily be detected by a dowser. Basically mineral extract resonances are activated by applying a high electric field to them. Some users have found they work well for them. Others have found they feel worse when a RadiTech is on in the building they are in. We suggest that you get one on approval.

RayMaster

RayMaster SP1 is a pyramid and SP2 is a small rectangular plastic box. The manufacturers claim that it compensates for the damaging influence of the electrosmog which now surrounds us. It is meant to help your body cells 'work optimally'. The following effects are claimed to be removed or significantly helped: fatigue, nervousness, allergies, neurodermatitis, asthma, somnipathy (troubled sleep), sterility, heart-rhythm disturbances, depression, lack of concentration, etc.

It is passive, without a battery, relying on incoming electromagnetic radiation to energise its resonances. Inside, it consists of some glass tubes with wire coiled around them in an unusual pattern and two of the tubes are filled with a mixed metallic powder. These devices certainly will have some electromagnetic resonances and therefore some influence.

However the power in any signals that they generate will be tiny, and our confidence is not enhanced by the pseudo-scientific gobble-de-gook text that we have been sent to encourage us to purchase them.

Sevenstar International Energy Balancer

The distributor claims that this gives people a natural resistance to the effects of TV and computer monitors, static electricity and earth rays. All its powers seem to be based around the number 7 rather than any electromagnetic properties.

Spiral of Tranquillity

There are several (moulded spiral, pendant and keyring) gemstone-based 'energy balancers' for home, car and personal use. They were originally devised, on the basis of historical research, intuition and dowsing over 25 years by Clive Beadon. When he died a few years ago they were taken over by Michael Poynder. There is no currently known electromagnetic basis for these working but many people are apparently delighted with the change they brought to their lives. (01929 480 735)

Takionic products

There is a wide range of Takionic products (belts, headbands, simple beads, fancy jewellery, massage oil, mattresses) ranging in price from about £20 to £1500.

Their patented complex high-tech material known as Optimum Resonant Material (ORM) has resonances in the 4 to 16 micron (μm) range, which is in the far-infra-red region of the spectrum. If this is truly the case then it is associated with heating effects and may well have a solid physical basis of interacting with human body energies.

Tele-puter Beacon

These and other devices are used by London-based 'harmoniser', Jacqui Beacon (0181 455 7912). She and a colleague balance energies in a building using various resonant coloured mineral based glass items. We have heard of some very satisfied customers but have no personal experience of their work.

Tecno AO

"**Tecno AO** offer small devices which attach to your VDU or mobile phone and emit a constant alpha wave at a similar strength to that of a human brain in certain states of non-activity. This in turn helps to stabilise the electromagnetic structures within the body and enables them to resist the disturbance from random radiations." So reads one of the leaflets we have seen.

We have been trialling a Tecno AO device on a computer and believe it might be having some beneficial effects. It is not 'directly powered', instead it picks up its energy from the computer monitor scan fields or mobile phone microwaves. I am at a loss to see how it might be working, though, as the fields its resonances are said to put out are tiny (0.15 picotesla). Even the Earth's Schumann resonances (natural EMFs that have always existed and that we have been exposed to in the course of our planetary and species evolution), are about 200 times higher than the Tecno AO signals.

Their literature claims they are of the same order as human brain wave signals. Maybe they are, but to suggest that you can generate these tiny levels at a distance from the brain and they will somehow manage to get themselves across the distance and into the brain at a level which will affect it, seems less likely. My science tells me rationally that these devices cannot be effective at these signal levels, even invoking stochastic resonance phenomena.

Research carried out at Cochin Hospital (Paris) has shown almost a 25% reduction in stress, a 13% increase in VDU operator speed, and improvement in concentration and alertness of 23% and 9% respectively. Follow-up questionnaires showed improvement in, or disappearance of, a wide range of health problems often attributed to other causes.

A recent double-blind study at Southampton Health Authority (by Derek Clement-Croome from Reading University and consultant John Jukes) showed similar improvements. Their 1999 study showed that in any four working weeks, 50% of staff in a typical office equipped with computers experienced between seven and 12 symptoms of headaches, dry itchy eyes, tiredness and fatigue, aching backs, necks and limbs, rashes, coughs and sneezes, depression, irritability and loss of concentration and memory.

One hundred people working in separate wings at the offices of Southampton and South West Hampshire Health Authority were involved in the study. Techno AO devices, which sit on top of the computer screen, were given to 50 staff working in one wing for a month, while the rest received a dummy.

Then the devices were switched round, but no one knew which were real and which fake until the results were recorded at the end of the study. When the real devices were operating, the number of symptoms fell by between 27% and 44%, with an average reduction of 36%. As soon as they were taken away, the symptom level shot up again.

UT Code software

This claims to work using Unified Field Theory and, once loaded on your personal computer, it decreases the tendency towards chaos and therefore decreases stress and improves your health and well-being. The promoters also claim that it enhances the performance of electronics systems. Having designed both computer hardware and software systems I do not believe their claims are based in our reality.

VDU screens

Modern VDUs (Computer Monitors) do not benefit significantly from screens in terms of reducing electromagnetic fields. They can be useful to reduce any reflections of windows or lights. They are only intended for use with normal cathode-ray tube (TV) type of displays.

Cheaper screens usually only can reduce glare and reflections and/or enhance contrast.

More expensive screens (typically over £75) have an earth wire attached and, when correctly installed, these greatly reduce any electric fields coming from the monitor. However most modern VDUs are 'Low radiation' *(MPRII or TCO92 or TCO95 compliant - see label on rear of the VDU to check this)* and they give off virtually no electric fields due to their design.

If you are very sensitive to electromagnetic radiation then the best type of screen to use, by far, are the new flat screen TFT displays. These are clear, bright and virtually flicker and EMF free, though they do cost more than an equivalent standard VDU.

Vortex unit

This is a unit designed to remove geopathic and electropathic stress from a house. We have no personal experience of this unit and have heard both good and bad reports from people who have purchased one. The person who devised it is a good bio-physicist who has spent many years investigating the harmful effects of electromagnetic fields on people and animals.

CHAPTER EIGHT
USEFUL INFORMATION

The writers of this book, and the other services offered by them:-

A & J Philips,
2, Tower Road, Sutton, Ely, Cambs.
CB6 2QA.
Tel: 0897 100 800
(Premium rate line @ £1.50 per minute)
Web Page: http://www.powerwatch.org.uk/

- Hire of meters measuring electric and magnetic fields.
- Hire of meters measuring microwave emissions from mobile phone masts - ask for availablility.
- Advice and information helpline: 0897 100 800 for your individual circumstances.
- Advice and information about **mobile phones** and their **masts.**
- Advice and information about pylons and substations.
- Consultancy service for residential and business premises.
- Demand switches.
- Living wih Electricity (2nd edition, 1997), £12.00 including p&p

---

Retailers of monitors for the detection and measurement of Electromagnetic radiation ELF, VLF, RF and MICROWAVE

Perspective Scientific Limited, 100, Baker Street, London. W1M 1LA
Tel: 0171 486 6837 Fax: 0171 487 3023
Email: service@perspective.co.uk
web Page: http://www.demon.co.uk/radiation-instruments/

Surveyor with a particular interest in properties with EMF issues.
John Meredith, Chartered Surveyor,
Tel: 0171 589 3443

Surveyor specialising in wayleave issues.
Colin Gell, Seraph Surveying Services,
Tel: 0115 962 2888

Liaison person for British campaigns against the erection of mobile phone base masts.
Clive Hicklin, Tel: 01752 362434 (after 5.30 p.m.)

Microwave detectors (for monitoring microwave ovens)
The Microlarm,
available from:
The Natural Collection, PO Box 2111, Bath, BA1 2ZQ.
Tel: 01225 442288

Neutralising undersheets for beds.
available from:
Natural Therapeutics, 25, New Road, Spalding, Lincolnshire
PE11 1DQ

Building for a Future - a quarterly magazine, published for the Association for Environment-Conscious Building.
Enquiries to:
The Editor, 'Building for a Future', Nant-y-Garreg, Saron, Llandysul, Carmarthenshire SA44 5EJ
Tel/Fax: 01559 370908
Email: editor.bff@aecb.net
Web: http://www.aecb.net/magazine

The Healthy House - a mail order company specialising in equipment to combat allergies
The Healthy House, Cold Harbour, Ruscombe, Stroud, Gloucestershire.
GL6 6DA
Tel: 01453 752216 Fax: 01453 753533
Web: http://www.healthy-house.co.uk

Centre for Alternative Technology, Llwyngwern Quarry, Machynlleth, Powys, Wales. SY20 9AZ
- "a unique demonstration centre designed to inspire, inform and enable society to move towards ecologically sustainable lifestyles"
Tel: 01654 702400
Fax: 01654 702782
email: info@cat.org.uk
Web: http//:www.cat.org.uk

London Hazards Centre, Interchange Studios, Dalby Street, London, NW5 3NQ.
Produces a newsletter and factsheets on all types of hazards, especially health and safety issues at work.
Tel: 0171 267 3387
Fax: 0171 267 3397
Email: lonhaz@mcr1.poptel.org.uk
Web: http://www.lhc.org.uk

For people who are Electrically Sensitive, there is an excellent support service and source of information.
The Association for the Electrically and VDT-injured.
P.O. Box 15126, 10465 Stockholm, Sweden.
Web: http://www.feb.se/
The publications are available in English.

Recommended Reading

Biological Effects of Electromagnetic Fields - C. Polk & E. Postow, CRC Press, inc. New York (ISBN 0-8493-0641-8)

Cross Currents - Robert Becker, 1990, Los Angeles. Tarcher

Electromagnetic Man - Smith & Best (1989). Unfortunately out of print since 1992. Very good and well worth reading, if you can get a copy from your local library.

H is for EcoHome - Anna Kruger, published by Gaia Books Ltd., 66, Charlotte Street, London W1P 1LR (ISBN 1-85675-030-2)

Living wih Electricity (2nd edition), available at £12.00 including p&p, from A & J Philips (ISBN 0-95245-031-3) (address above)

Melatonin Your Body's Natural Wonder Drug - Russel J Reiter, Bantam Books, London (ISBN 0-553-10017-3)

Something in the Air - Roger Coghill
Available directly from: 01495 763 389

Super Health - Dr Mark Payne, 1992, Thorsons, London.
(ISBN 0-7225-2589-3)

V.D.U. Work and the Hazards to Health - London Hazards Centre, Interchange Studios, Dalby Street, London, NW5 3NQ.
Tel. 0171 267 3387   (ISBN 0 948974 11 7)

Details of **Electromagnetics Hazard & Therapy** newsletter available from Information Production Services, PO Box 2039, Shoreham by Sea, BN43 5JD.

Websites

http://www.powerwatch.org.uk/

http://www.cogreslab.demon.co.uk/

http://www.demon.co.uk/radiation-instruments/

http://www2.cruzio.com:80/~rbedard/emflinks.html

http://www.tassie.net.au/emfacts/enzine.html

http://www.microwavenews.com/index.html

http://www.milligauss.com/

http://www.ncf.carleton.ca/bridlewood-emfinfo/

http://www.bemi.se/

http://www.feb.se/

http://www.feb.se/EMF-L/EMF-L.html

http://www2.cruzio.com/~rbedard/whatsnew.html

http://members.cruzio.com/~rbedard/WaveGuid.html

http://www.epsilon-ltd.co.uk/emht

The NIEHS Working Group report which came out in 1998 which classified power frequency EMFs as possible human carcinogens (available free from NIEHS web site) at:
http://www.niehs.nih.gov/emfrapid/home.htm

APPENDICES

Appendix One

We have used nanotesla as the main unit throughout the book, adding measurements in microtesla where this has seemed to be appropriate. There are 1000 nanotesla (nT) to one microtesla (µT).

Electricity Companies and the NRPB often use microtesla as thier main unit. This may not necessarily mean that they want field levels to look as low as they can (!), but because most risk assessments they make are to do with the thermal effects of EMFs which they measure at high levels. Recent laboratory studies have shown that cells produce heat shock proteins (as if they had been heated) at *very* low EMF levels, but this research is at a very early stage and we do not know what the implications of this might be.

Another unit of measurement, used especially in the U.S., though also used by some measuring equipment available in this country (often imported) is Gauss (G). There are 100 µT in one Gauss.

In the table below m = milli, µ = micro, n = nano. Milli = 1/1000 of the unit e.g. 1mG = 1/1000 Gauss, 1µG = 1/1000 mG, 1nG = 1/1000 µG

Nanotesla	Microtesla	Gauss
1 nT	0.001µT	10µG
10 nT	0.01µT	0.1mG
100 nT	0.1µT	1 mG
1,000 nT	1 µT	10 mG
10,000 nT	10 µT	100 mG

Appendix Two

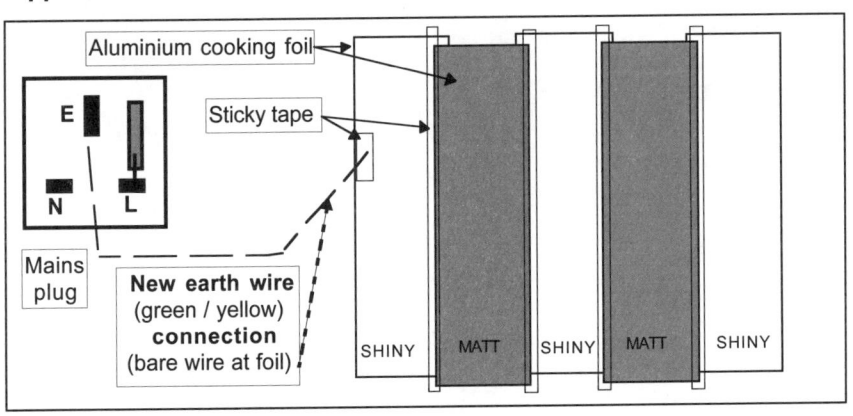